Analysis of
FRACTIONAL
STOCHASTIC
PROCESSES
Advances and Applications

7th Jagna International Workshop

Analysis of

FRACTIONAL STOCHASTIC PROCESSES

Advances and Applications

Jagna, Bohol, Philippines   6 – 9 January 2014

Editors

Christopher C Bernido
M Victoria Carpio-Bernido

Research Center for Theoretical Physics, Central Visayan Institute Foundation, Philippines

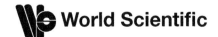 **World Scientific**

NEW JERSEY • LONDON • SINGAPORE • BEIJING • SHANGHAI • HONG KONG • TAIPEI • CHENNAI

Published by

World Scientific Publishing Co. Pte. Ltd.

5 Toh Tuck Link, Singapore 596224

USA office: 27 Warren Street, Suite 401-402, Hackensack, NJ 07601

UK office: 57 Shelton Street, Covent Garden, London WC2H 9HE

Library of Congress Cataloging-in-Publication Data
Jagna International Workshop (7th : 2014 : Jagna, Bohol, Philippine)
 Analysis of fractional stochastic processes : advances and applications : 7th Jagna International Workshop, Jagna, Bohol, Philippine, 6–9 January 2014 / editors, Christopher C. Bernido, M. Victoria Carpio-Bernido, Research Center for Theoretical Physics, Central Visayan Institute Foundation, Philippines.
  pages cm
 Includes bibliographical references and indexes.
 ISBN 978-9814618342 (hardcover : alk. paper)
 1. Stochastic processes--Congresses. 2. Fractional differential equations--Congresses. I. Bernido, Christopher C. (Christopher Caseñas), editor. II. Carpio-Bernido, M. Victoria, editor. III. Central Visayan Institute Foundation. Research Center for Theoretical Physics, organizer. IV. Title. V. Title: 7th Jagna International Workshop : Analysis of fractional stochastic processes : advances and applications.
 QC20.7.S8J34 2014
 519.2'3--dc23

                         2014039633

British Library Cataloguing-in-Publication Data
A catalogue record for this book is available from the British Library.

Printed in Singapore

CONTENTS

Complex Social Systems

Fractional Quantum Mechanics

Macromolecules and Cells

7th Jagna International Workshop (2014)
International Journal of Modern Physics: Conference Series
Vol. 36 (2015) 1502001 (7 pages)
© The Authors
DOI: 10.1142/S2010194515020012

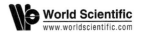

Preface

Stochastic processes with memory are the focus of intensive mathematical, experimental, and computational studies due to the widening spectrum of applications in natural and social sciences. To engage more in these exciting new developments, the Research Center for Theoretical Physics (RCTP), Central Visayan Institute Foundation, organized the 7th Jagna International Workshop: Analysis of Fractional Stochastic Processes: Advances and Applications on 6–9 January 2014. The Workshop aimed to discuss (a) novel vis-à-vis standard approaches in fractional stochastic analysis; (b) experimental and theoretical highlights in applications to nanotechnology, mass rapid transit systems, critical transitions in economic systems, fractional quantum mechanics, polymer physics, among others; and (c) challenges, recent breakthroughs and open questions. The informal nature of the Workshop held in the coastal town of Jagna in the island province of Bohol, Philippines, was essentially meant to foster active interaction among speakers and participants so that possible research targets could be clearly defined.

The papers in this volume serve as a record of (i) review and pedagogical lectures given with graduate students and young Ph.D.'s as the target audience, and (ii) new research results. As in previous workshops of the series, camera-ready manuscripts were contributed by lecturers and speakers for the publication of the Proceedings to allow a wider audience to benefit from the Workshop.

The Workshop organizers wish to express their gratitude to the speakers, lecturers, and participants, as well as to the Workshop sponsors for the invaluable support. They are also grateful to the Workshop project assistants and staff who ensured the smooth running of the Workshop.

C. C. Bernido and M. V. Carpio-Bernido
Editors

WORKSHOP SPONSORS

The organizers are grateful to:

Philippine Long Distance Telephone Company (PLDT) — SMART Foundation; SMART Communications, Inc.; Abdus Salam International Centre for Theoretical Physics; Alexander von Humboldt Foundation; Mindanao State University — Iligan Institute of Technology; Governor Edgardo M. Chatto, Province of Bohol; Mayor Fortunato R. Abrenilla, Municipality of Jagna.

WORKSHOP ORGANIZERS

Christopher C. Bernido and M. Victoria Carpio-Bernido
Research Center for Theoretical Physics
Central Visayan Institute Foundation
Jagna, Bohol 6308, Philippines

WORKSHOP PROJECT ASSISTANTS
Central Visayan Institute Foundation
Faculty and Staff

Maria Johanna B. Bagaipo, Rey A. Aceron, Maria Julie Pearl B. Aclan, Noel B. Acasio, Arlyn S. Aceron, Victor S. Bucog, Jeric G. Daguplo, Diosdada F. Cagas, Maria Mae S. Cagas, Raymond S. Cruel, Geneliza A. Galope, Vicencia B. Galbizo, Pablita C. Galos, Mae Donna P. Licaros, Ruby Anna O. Rañoa, Janice P. Tutor, Maricar S. Acenas, Alma Gilbretta T. Bolinas, Jonalizae P. Cuñado, Aisa S. Timbal, Annabeth Q. Acedo, Noel D. Romero, Victor G. Daguplo.

List of participants

Arnold C. Alguno
Physics Department
MSU-Iligan Institute of Technology
Iligan City 9200, Philippines
email: arnold.alguno@g.msuiit.edu.ph

Henry P. Aringa
Physics Department
Mindanao State University
Marawi City, Philippines
email: henparinga@yahoo.com

Rommel G. Bacabac
Medical Biophysics Group
Physics Department
University of San Carlos, Talamban,
Cebu City, Philippines
email: rgbacabac@gmail.com

Wilson I. Barredo
Physics Department
MSU-Iligan Institute of Technology
Bonifacio Avenue, Tibanga
9200 Iligan City, Philippines
email: barredo1234@yahoo.com

Christopher C. Bernido
Research Center for Theoretical Physics
Central Visayan Institute Foundation
Jagna, Bohol 6308, Philippines
email: cbernido@mozcom.com

Corazon C. Bernido
Philippine Nuclear Research Institute
Commonwealth Ave., Diliman
Quezon City, Philippines
email: cber823@yahoo.com

Jinky B. Bornales
Physics Department
MSU-Iligan Institute of Technology
Iligan City 9200, Philippines
email: jbornales@gmail.com

Cresente Cabahug
Physics Department
MSU-Iligan Institute of Technology
Iligan City 9200, Philippines

M. Victoria Carpio-Bernido
Research Center for Theoretical Physics
Central Visayan Institute Foundation
Jagna, Bohol 6308, Philippines
email: cbernido@mozcom.com

Mark Nolan P. Confesor
Physics Department
MSU-Iligan Institute of Technology
Iligan City 9200, Philippines
email: marknolan2006@gmail.com

Raymond S. Cruel
Central Visayan Institute Foundation
Jagna, Bohol 6308, Philippines

Jonalizae P. Cuñado
Central Visayan Institute Foundation
Jagna, Bohol 6308, Philippines

Matthew George O. Escobido
W. Sycip Graduate School of Business
Asian Institute of Management

123 Paseo de Roxas Ave.
Makati City 1260, Philippines
email: mescobido@aim.edu

Jose Perico Esguerra
National Institute of Physics
University of the Philippines
Diliman, Quezon City 1101, Philippines
email: perry.esguerra@gmail.com

Vicencia B. Galbizo
Central Visayan Institute Foundation
Jagna, Bohol 6308, Philippines

Geneliza A. Galope
Central Visayan Institute Foundation
Jagna, Bohol 6308, Philippines

Pablita C. Galos
Central Visayan Institute Foundation
Jagna, Bohol 6308, Philippines

Beverly V. Gemao
Physics Department
MSU-Iligan Institute of Technology
Iligan City 9200, Philippines

Mary Ann Go
Department of Quantum Science
Research School of Physics
and Engineering Australian
National University
Canberra, Australia
email: maryann.go@anu.edu.au

Ferdinand Jamil
Mathematics Department
MSU-Iligan Institute of Technology
Iligan City 9200, Philippines

Roger Joseph Lacubtan
Physics Department
MSU-Iligan Institute of Technology
Bonifacio Avenue, Tibanga
9200 Iligan City, Philippines

Angie Laure
Physics Department

MSU-Iligan Institute of Technology
Bonifacio Avenue, Tibanga
9200 Iligan City, Philippines

Swee Cheng Lim
Faculty of Engineering
Multimedia University Malaysia
Jalan Multimedia,
63100 Cyberjaya, Selangor, Malaysia
email: sclim47@gmail.com

Sheila Menchavez
Mathematics Department
MSU-Iligan Institute of Technology
Iligan City 9200, Philippines

Ralf Metzler
Institute for Physics & Astronomy
University of Potsdam
Potsdam, Germany
and Department of Physics
Tampere University of Technology
Tampere, Finland
email: rmetzler@uni-potsdam.de
and ralf.metzler@tut.fi

Christopher P. Monterola
Complex Systems Group
Computing Science Department
Institute of High Performance
Computing (IHPC),
Fusionopolis, 1 Fusionopolis Way
#16-16 Connexis, 138632 Singapore
email: monterolac@ihpc.a-star.edu.sg

Sithi V. Muniandy
Department of Physics
University of Malaya
50603 Kuala Lumpur,Malaysia
email: msithi@um.edu.my

Mary Madelynn Nayga
National Institute of Physics
University of the Philippines
Diliman, Quezon City 1101, Philippines
email: mnayga@nip.upd.edu.ph

Harvey Niere
Department of Economics
Mindanao State University
9700 Marawi City, Philippines
email: hmniere@gmail.com

Ruby Anna O. Rañoa
Central Visayan Institute Foundation
Jagna, Bohol 6308, Philippines
email: rubyanna_ranoa@yahoo.com

Deivid Rioferio
Public Affairs Group
Smart Communications, Inc.
Smart Tower, 6799 Ayala Avenue
Makati City, Philippines
email: dbrioferio@smart.com.ph

Jerome Sadudaquil
Department of Physical Sciences
and Mathematics
University of the Philippines
Taft Avenue, Manila, Philippines
email: jeromesadudaquil@rocketmail.com

James Salig, Jr.
Misamis University
H. T. Feliciano St., 7200
Ozamiz City, Philippines
email: jamesboss2@gmail.com

Jan Philippe B. Sambo
Physics Department
MSU-Iligan Institute of Technology
Bonifacio Avenue, Tibanga
9200 Iligan City, Philippines
email: japhisam@gmail.com

Ma. Esther O. Santos
PLDT-Smart Foundation, Inc.
7th Floor Ramon Cojuangco Building
Makati Avenue corner dela Rosa St.,
Makati City, Philippines

Georgiy Shevchenko
Department of Mechanics
and Mathematics
Taras Shevchenko National
University of Kyiv, Volodymyrska 64
01601 Kiev, Ukraine
email: zhoraster@gmail.com

José Luís da Silva
Centro de Ciencias Matemáticas
University of Madeira
P 9000-390 Funchal, Madeira, Portugal
email: luis@uma.pt

Ludwig Streit
BiBoS, Universität Bielefeld
33615 Bielefeld, Germany
and Centro de Ciencias Matemáticas
University of Madeira, P 9000-390
Funchal, Madeira, Portugal
email: streit@pcserv.physik.uni-
bielefeld.de

Herry P. Suryawan
Department of Mathematics
Sanata Dharma University
Yogyakarta, Indonesia
email: herrypribs@usd.ac.id

Jeffrey Tare
National Institute of Physics
University of the Philippines
Diliman, Quezon City 1101, Philippines
email: jeffreytare@gmail.com

Janice Tutor
Central Visayan Institute Foundation
Jagna, Bohol 6308, Philippines

Dominador Vaso
Physics Department
MSU-Iligan Institute of Technology
Bonifacio Avenue, Tibanga
Iligan City 9200, Philippines

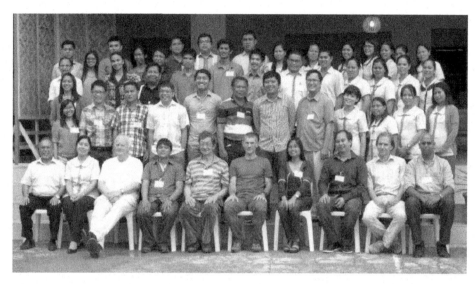

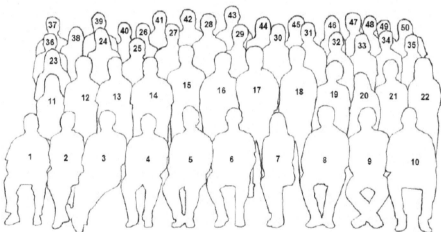

1. Christopher C. Bernido; 2. M. Victoria Carpio-Bernido; 3. Ludwig Streit; 4. Rommel G Bacabac; 5. Swee Cheng Lim; 6. José Luís da Silva; 7. Jinky B. Bornales; 8. Christopher P. Monterola; 9. Georgiy Shevchenko; 10. Sithi V. Muniandy; 11. Mary Madelynn I. Nayga; 12. Ferdinand Jamil; 13. Wilson Barredo; 14. Harvey Niere; 15. James B. Salig, Jr.; 16. Henry P. Aringa; 17. Mark Nolan P. Confesor; 18. Matthew G. O. Escobido; 19. Maria Johanna B. Bagaipo; 20. Ruby Anna O. Rañoa; 21. Jonalizae P. Cuñado; 22. Vicencia B. Galbizo; 23. Mary Ann Go; 24. Beverly V. Gemao; 25. Jose Perico Esguerra; 26. Cresente Cabahug; 27. Roger Joseph Lacubtan; 28. Dominador Vaso; 29. Jerome A. Sadudaquil; 30. Raymond S. Cruel; 31. Noel B. Acasio; 32. Maricar S. Acenas; 33. Maria Mae S. Cagas; 34. Arlyn S. Aceron; 35. Aisa S. Timbal; 36. Arnold C. Alguno; 37. Jeffrey Tare; 38. Sheila Menchavez; 39. Jan Philippe B. Sambo; 40. Angie Laure; 41. Rey A. Aceron; 42. Herry P. Suryawan; 43. Jeric G. Daguplo; 44. Alma Gilbretta T. Bolinas; 45. Mae Donna P. Licaros; 46. Geneliza A. Galope; 47. Pablita C. Galos; 48. Janice P. Tutor; 49. Annabeth Q. Acedo; 50. Diosdada F. Cagas.

WORKSHOP PROGRAMME

TIME	January 6, Monday	January 7, Tuesday	January 8, Wednesday	January 9, Thursday
8:30 – 9:30	*REGISTRATION*	S. C. Lim, "Some fractional and multifractional processes and their possible applications"	J. L. da Silva, "Asymptotic scaling for double intersection penalized Brownian motion - A white noise approach"	8-00 FREE DAY DISCUSSIONS and / or TOUR
	(9:00) WELCOME SESSION			
9:30 – 10:00	COFFEE BREAK	COFFEE BREAK	COFFEE BREAK	
10:00 – 11:00	L. Streit, "Fractional Brownian motion and polymers: Learning from each other"	S. V. Muniandy, "Fractional dynamics of carrier transport in disordered organic semiconductors"	G. Shevchenko, "Adapted representations in fractional and mixed models: with applications"	
	J. B. Bornales, "Self-repelling fractional Brownian motion – the case of higher order self-intersections"			
11:00 – 12:00	J. P. Sambo, "Fractional Brownian modeled linear polymer chains with one dimensional Metropolis Monte Carlo simulation"	C. P. Monterola, "Modeling urban dynamics: A complex systems approach"	C. C. Bernido, "Path summation with memory" (30 min)	
			H. P. Suryawan, "Topics in fractional path integrals" (30 min)	
12:00 – 13:30	LUNCH	LUNCH	LUNCH	
13:30 – 14:15	R. G. Bacabac, "Probing the mechanics of molecules and cells with optical tweezers"	F. W. Wiegel, "A stochastic model for early AIDS infection"	M. G. O. Escobido, "Critical slowing down in a dynamic duopoly"	
14:15 – 14:30	W. Barredo, "On the diffusion of alpha-helical proteins in solvents"			
14:30 – 15:00	M. N. P. Confesor, "Fluctuation theorems in soft matter systems"	M. A. Go, "Four-dimensional photostimulation: Stimulating neurons in space and time"	H. Niere, "Measuring efficiency of international crude oil market: a multifractality approach"	
15:00 – 15:30	COFFEE BREAK	GROUP PHOTO / COFFEE BREAK	COFFEE BREAK	
15:30 – 15:50	J. Tare, "Space fractional Schrödinger equation for a quadrupolar triple Dirac δ-potential"	R. Metzler, "Non-ergodicity and ageing in anomalous diffusion processes" (by Skype)	Roundtable Discussion CLOSING	
15:50 – 16:10	M. M. Nayga, "Lévy path integral approach to the fractional Schrödinger equation with δ-perturbed infinite square well"			
16:10 – 16:30	R. J. Lacubtan, "Robust method for trapping self-propelling particles"			
16:30 – 17:15	Tutorial Lecture I: G. Shevchenko, "Fractional Brownian motion in a nutshell"	Tutorial Lecture II: G. Shevchenko, "Fractional Brownian motion in a nutshell"		
19:00	WELCOME DINNER			

7th Jagna International Workshop (2014)
International Journal of Modern Physics: Conference Series
Vol. 36 (2015) 1560001 (14 pages)
© The Authors
DOI: 10.1142/S2010194515600010

Some fractional and multifractional Gaussian processes: A brief introduction

S. C. Lim

Faculty of Engineering, Multimedia University
63100 Cyberjaya, Selangor Darul Ehsan, Malaysia
sclim47@gmail.com

C. H. Eab

Department of Chemistry, Faculty of Science
Chulalongkorn University, Bangkok 10330, Thailand
Chaihok.E@chula.ac.th

Published 2 January 2015

This paper gives a brief introduction to some important fractional and multifractional Gaussian processes commonly used in modelling natural phenomena and man-made systems. The processes include fractional Brownian motion (both standard and the Riemann-Liouville type), multifractional Brownian motion, fractional and multifractional Ornstein-Uhlenbeck processes, fractional and mutifractional Reisz-Bessel motion. Possible applications of these processes are briefly mentioned.

Keywords: Fractional and multifractional stochastic processes; locally self-similarity; short and long-range dependence.

PACS Numbers: 02.50.-r, 02.50.Ey, 05.40.-a

1. Introduction

During the past few decades, fractional calculus[1–4] has found applications in diverse fields ranging from physical and biological sciences, engineering to internet traffic and economics. One of the main reasons for its popularity in modelling many phenomena is that it provides a natural setting for describing processes which are fractal in nature and with memory.[5–11] Many applications of fractional calculus are based on the fractional integro-differential equations.[12–15] For example, various types of fractional diffusion equations and fractional Langevin-type equations have been proposed to model anomalous diffusion, and both deterministic and stochastic fractional equations are used to describe viscoelastic phenomena, telecommunication, and other systems in science and engineering.[16–29]

The usual way to obtain concrete realization of a particular fractional model is to associate it with a fractional generalization of an ordinary stochastic process. This can be carried out nicely due to the smooth integration of fractional calculus and probability theory. The most well-known among these fractional stochastic processes include fractional Brownian motion[30–32] and fractional Levy motion.[33–35] Another fractional stochastic process of interest is fractional Ornstein-Uhlenbeck process.[36–38]

Fractional Brownian motion (FBM) and fractional Ornstein-Uhlenbeck (FOU) process are characterized by a single parameter. It is possible to extend FBM to bifractional Brownian motion[39] and mixed FBM,[40] which are indexed by two parameters and two or more parameters respectively. Similarly, FOU process can also be generalized to a process parametrized by two fractional indices.[41, 42] Other examples of stochastic processes with two indices are fractional Riesz-Bessel motion (FRBM)[43, 44] and Gaussian process with generalized Cauchy covariance (generalized Cauchy process).[45, 46] In general, processes parametrized by two indices can provide more flexibility in modelling physical phenomena. In the case of the generalized Cauchy process both have the advantage that the two indices provide separate characterization of the fractal dimension or self-similar property, a local property, and the long-range dependence, a global property. This is in contrast to models based on fractional Brownian motion which characterize these two properties with a single parameter. On the other hand, the two indices of FRBM characterize the long-range dependence and intermittency separately. In contrast, FBM is not intermittent.

Further generalization of fractional process can be carried out by replacing the constant index by a continuous function of time. In this way, one obtains multifractional Brownian motion[47, 48] and multifractional Ornstein-Uhlenbeck process.[49] Similarly, it is possible to have the multifractional extension of Riesz-Bessel motion[50, 51] and generalized Cauchy process. These processes can be used to describe systems with variable fractal dimension and variable memory. In this short paper we shall restrict our discussion on some fractional and multifractional Gaussian processes, and mentioned briefly their possible applications. The non-Gaussian fractional and multifractional Levy motion will not be considered here.

2. Fractional Brownian Motion

Among all the fractional stochastic processes applied to modeling natural and man-made systems, fractional Brownian motion (FBM) can be regarded as the most widely used. Here we would like to summarise briefly the main properties of FBM.

The standard FBM as introduced by Mandelbrot and Van Ness[52] is defined by the following moving average representation:

$$D_H(t) = \frac{1}{\Gamma(H+1/2)} \left\{ \int_{-\infty}^{0} \left[(t-u)^{H-1/2} - (-u)^{H-1/2} \right] dB(u) \right.$$

$$\left. + \int_{0}^{t} (t-u)^{H-1/2} dB(u) \right\}, \tag{1}$$

where $B(t)$ is the standard Brownian motion, Γ is the gamma function and the Hölder exponent (or Hurst index) H lies in the range $0 < H < 1$. Equation (1) can be written more compactly as

$$B_H(t) = \frac{1}{\Gamma(H+1/2)} \int_{-\infty}^{\infty} \left[(t-u)_{+}^{H-1/2} - (-u_{+})^{H-1/2} \right] dB(u), \tag{2}$$

where $(x)_+ = \max(x, 0)$. Note that there exists an equivalent representation of FBM known as the harmonizable or the spectral representation:[33]

$$B_H(t) = \frac{1}{2\pi} \int_{-\infty}^{\infty} \frac{e^{it\xi} - 1}{|\xi|^{H+1/2}} dB(\xi). \tag{3}$$

B_H is a Gaussian process with zero mean and its variance and covariance are respectively

$$\left\langle \left(B_H(t) \right)^2 \right\rangle = \sigma_H^2 |t|^{2H}, \tag{4}$$

$$\left\langle \left(B_H(t) B_H(s) \right)^2 \right\rangle = \frac{\sigma_H^2}{2} \left[|t|^{2H} + |s|^{2H} - |t-s|^{2H} \right], \tag{5}$$

with

$$\sigma_H^2 = \left\langle \left(B_H(1) \right)^2 \right\rangle = \frac{\Gamma(1-2H)\cos(\pi H)}{\pi H}. \tag{6}$$

FBM defined above is continuous everywhere non-differentiable with an unique scaling exponent H, a characteristic of a monofractal process.

The standard FBM B_H has some desirable properties. It is a self-similar process of order H:

$$B_H(at) = a^H B_H(t), \qquad\qquad \forall a > 0, \quad t \in \mathbb{R}, \tag{7}$$

where the equality is in the sense of finite joint distributions. Though B_H is itself non-stationary, its increment process

$$\Delta B_H(t, \tau) \equiv B_H(t+\tau) - B_H(t), \qquad\qquad \tau > 0, \tag{8}$$

is stationary with covariance

$$\left\langle \Delta B_H(t, \tau_1) \Delta B_H(t, \tau_2) \right\rangle = \frac{\sigma_H^2}{2} \left[|\tau_1|^{2H} + |\tau_2|^{2H} - |\tau_1 - \tau_2|^{2H} \right]. \tag{9}$$

Self-similarity together with stationary increments imply

$$B_H(t+\tau) - B(t) = a^{-H}\big[B_H(t+a\tau) - B_H(t)\big], \qquad \forall a > 0, \quad t \in \mathbb{R}. \tag{10}$$

In contrast to the local properties which depend mainly on the correlations between points that are close to each other, the long and short-range dependence of a stochastic process is a global property that measures the total strength of the correlation over a large domain. Given a Gaussian stochastic process $Y(t)$ with correlation $R(t, s) = \big\langle Y(s)Y(t) \big\rangle \Big[\big\langle (Y(s))^2 \big\rangle \big\langle (Y(t))^2 \big\rangle\Big]^{-1/2}$ we say that it has long-range dependence (LRD) or long memory if the integral $\int_{\mathbb{R}} R(t, t+u)du$ is divergent. On the other hand, if the integral is convergent, the process has short-range dependence (SRD) or short memory.[37] One can easily verify that FBM is LRD except for $H = 1/2$, which corresponds to Brownian motion, a Markov process.

Despite the nice properties mentioned above, the standard FBM does not represent a causal time-invariant system as there does exist a well-defined impulse response function. There is another type of FBM, the one-sided FBM first introduced by Barnes and Allan[53] using the Riemann-Liouville (RL) fractional integral:

$$X_H(t) = \frac{1}{\Gamma(H+1/2)} \int_0^t (t-u)^{H-1/2} dB(u), \tag{11}$$

represents a linear system driven by white noise $\eta(t)$, with the impulse response function $t^{H-1/2}/(\Gamma(H+1/2))$. The RL-FBM $X_H(t)$ is a zero-mean Gaussian process with a complicated covariance:

$$\big\langle X_H(t)X_H(s) \big\rangle = \frac{t^{H-1/2}s^{H+1/2}}{(H+1/2)\big(\Gamma(H+1/2)\big)^2} \, {}_2F_1\big(1, 1/2 - H, 3/2 + H, s/t\big), \tag{12}$$

where $s < t$ and ${}_2F_1$ is the Gauss hypergeometric function. However, the variance of X_H has the same time dependence as B_H:

$$\big\langle (X_H(t))^2 \big\rangle = \frac{t^{2H}}{2H\big(\Gamma(H+1/2)\big)^2}. \tag{13}$$

Except for the absence of stationary increments, X_H has many properties in common with B_H, such as self-similarity, regularity of sample path, LRD, etc. Absence of stationary property for its increments implies that X_H can not have a harmonizable representation, and it is also not possible to associate to X_H a generalized spectrum of power-law type as in the case of standard FBM. This is the main reason for the lesser use of FBM of RL-type in modeling systems with power law type spectrum. However, X_H has gained more popularity recently in some applications as the process is physically more realistic since it starts at time zero.

Applications of FBM are well-known and diverse. Here we just mention the more common ones such as anomalous transport phenomena in physical and biological sciences, telecommunication,[54] and finance.[30, 55]

3. Multifractional Brownian Motion

FBM can only be used in modelling phenomena which are monofractal with same irregularity globally and with constant memory as characterised by the constant Hölder exponent H. However, for real world systems global self-similarity seldom exists. Fixed scaling only holds for a certain finite range of intervals. In addition, empirical data indicate that the scaling exponent or order of self-similarity usually has more than one value. Thus in many complex heterogeneous systems there exist phenomena which exhibit multifractal properties with variable space and time dependent memory.[56–58] One simple way to generalize a mono-scaling FBM to a multi-scaling FBM (or multifractional Brownian motion, MBM) is to replace the constant Hölder exponent by $H(t), t \in \mathbb{R}^+$, a $(0,1)$-valued function with Hölder regularity $r, r > \sup H(t)$. In general $H(t)$ can be a deterministic or random function, and it needs not be a continuous function. This time-varying Hölder exponent $H(t)$ describes the local variations of the irregularity of the MBM. Such a generalization of FBM B_H to MBM $B_{H(t)}$ was carried out independently by Peltier and Lévy-Véhel[47] based on the moving-average representation and by Benassi *et al*[48] using the harmonizable representation. As expected, these two generalizations of MBM are almost certainly equivalent up to a multiplicative deterministic function of time.[59,60]

MBM does not satisfy the self-similar property and its increments are no longer stationary as a result of the time-dependence of the Hölder exponent. However, one expects $B_{H(t)}$ to behave like FBM locally. If an additional condition is imposed on $H(t)$ such that $H(t) \in C^r(\mathbb{R},(0,1)), t \in \mathbb{R}$ for some positive r with $r > \sup H(t)$, then it can be shown that $H(t_\circ)$ is almost certainly the Hölder exponent of the MBM at the point $t_\circ$; and the local Hausdorff and box dimensions of the graph of $B_{H(t)}$ at $t_\circ$ are almost certainly $2 - H(t_\circ)$. One can also characterize the above local fractal property by using the following notion. A process $Z(t)$ is said to satisfy the locally asymptotically self-similarity at a point $t_\circ$ if

$$\lim_{\rho \to 0+} \left[\frac{Z(t + \rho u) - Z(t_\circ)}{\rho^{H(t_\circ)}} \right]_{u \in \mathbb{R}} = \left(B_{H(t_\circ)}(u) \right)_{u \in \mathbb{R}}, \tag{14}$$

where the equality is up to a multiplicative deterministic function of time. It can be verified that $B_H(t)$ is locally asymptotically self-similar. Thus MBM at a time $t_\circ$ behaves locally like a FBM with Hölder exponent $H(t_\circ)$. Note that the time-dependent Hölder exponent has no effect on the long range dependence of the process. Just like FBM, $B_{H(t)}$ is a long memory process.

Similar to the case of standard FBM, one can also extend FBM of RL type to its corresponding multifractional process. By replacing H by $H(t)$ in (11), one gets MBM of RL type with the following covariance:[60,61]

$$\left\langle X_{H(s)} X_{H(t)} \right\rangle = \frac{{}_2F_1\left(1, \frac{1}{2} - H(t), H(s) + \frac{3}{2}, \frac{s}{t}\right)}{(2H(s) + 1)\Gamma\left(H(s) + \frac{1}{2}\right)\Gamma\left(H(t) + \frac{1}{2}\right)} s^{H(s) + \frac{1}{2}} t^{H(s) + \frac{1}{2}}. \tag{15}$$

The two types of MBM (standard and RL) have more properties in common as compared with the corresponding two types of FBM. They have non-stationary increments, and both are locally asymptotically self-similar with local fractal dimension at a point t_o given by $2 - H(t_o)$, and they are both LRD.

MBM has been applied to model many phenomena which have variable irregurities or variable memory. For example, it is used in modelling network traffic and signal processing,[62, 63] in geophysics for terrain modelling,[64, 65] in financial time series for stochastic volatility modelling,[66] and in modelling anomalous diffusion with variable memory.[67, 68]

Finally we remark that MBM can be further generalized. Various generalizations of MBM have been proposed[69, 70] to allow Hölder function to be very irregular, and enable the prescription of local intensity of jumps in space or time.

4. Fractional and Multifractional Ornstein-Uhlenbeck Process

FBM and MBM are used to model long memory phenomena. For describing systems which are short-range dependent, Ornstein-Uhlenbeck process can be a suitable candidate. Recall that Ornstein-Uhlenbeck process is the solution of the ordinary Langevin equation

$$D_t x(t) + \omega x(t) = \eta(t), \tag{16}$$

where $\eta(t)$ is standard white noise which can be regarded as the time derivative of Brownian motion in the sense of generalized function. Assuming $x(a) = 0$, the solution of (16) is given by

$$x(t) = \int_a^t e^{\omega(t-u)} \eta(u) du. \tag{17}$$

There are several ways to fractionalize Ornstein-Uhlenbeck process. One way is to replace the white noise by a fractional Gaussian noise in (16) or (17),[36, 37] or one can apply the Lamperti transformation to fractional Brownian motion.[37, 38]

In this paper we shall consider a different type of FOU processes. FOU process of Weyl type and Riemann-Liouville type can be defined as[71]

$$Y_\alpha^W(t) = \frac{1}{\Gamma(\alpha)} \int_{-\infty}^t (t-u)^{\alpha-1} e^{\omega(t-u)} \eta(u) du, \tag{18}$$

$$Y_\alpha^{RL}(t) = \frac{1}{\Gamma(\alpha)} \int_0^t (t-u)^{\alpha-1} e^{\omega(t-u)} \eta(u) du. \tag{19}$$

The condition $\alpha > 1/2$ is imposed to ensure finite variance for both the FOU processes. (18) and (19) can be regarded as the generalizations of (17), with $a = -\infty$ and $a = 0$. These fractional processes are solutions to the following nonlinear fractional Langevin equation:

$$\left(_a D_t + \omega\right)^\alpha Y(t) = \eta(t). \tag{20}$$

The Weyl fractional Ornstein-Uhlenbeck process $Y_\alpha^W(t)$ is stationary centred Gaussian process with variance and covariance

$$E\left(\left[Y_\alpha^W(t)\right]^2\right) = \frac{\Gamma(2\alpha - 1)(2\omega)^{1-2\alpha}}{\Gamma(\alpha)^2}, \tag{21a}$$

$$E\left(Y_\alpha^W(t)Y_\alpha^W(s)\right) = \frac{1}{\sqrt{\pi}\Gamma(\alpha)}\left(\frac{|t-s|}{2\omega}\right)^{\alpha-1/2}K_{\alpha-1/2}\left(\omega|t-s|\right), \quad t \neq s, \tag{21b}$$

where $K_\nu(z)$ is the modified Bessel function of second kind.[72] On the other hand, the Riemann-Liouville fractional Ornstein-Uhlenbeck process $Y_\alpha^{RL}(t)$ is a non-stationary centred Gaussian process with variance and covariance

$$E\left(\left[Y_\alpha^{RL}(t)\right]^2\right) = \frac{(2\omega)^{1-2\alpha}\gamma(2\alpha - 1, 2\omega t)}{\Gamma(\alpha)^2}, \tag{22a}$$

$$E\left(Y_\alpha^{RL}(t)Y_\alpha^{RL}(s)\right) = \frac{e^{-\omega(t+s)}s^\alpha t^{\alpha-1}}{\Gamma(\alpha+1)\Gamma(\alpha)}\Phi_1\left(1, 1-\alpha, 1+\alpha), \frac{s}{t}, 2\omega(s)\right), \quad t > s, \tag{22b}$$

where $\gamma(a, x)$ is the incomplete Gamma function, and $\Phi_1(a, b, c, x, y)$ is the confluent hypergeometric function in two variables. For discussion of properties and applications of the FOU process of Weyl and RL type, and their extension to FOU process with two indices can be found elsewhere.[41, 42, 71]

Just like the case of MBM, one can extend the two types of FOU processes to their corresponding multifractional OU (MOU) processes by replacing α by $\alpha(t)$. The covariance of the MOU process of Weyl type for $s < t$ is given by

$$E\left(Y_{\alpha(t)}^W(t)Y_{\alpha(s)}^W(s)\right) = \frac{e^{-\omega(t+s)}}{\Gamma(\alpha(t))\Gamma(\alpha(s))}\int_{-\infty}^s (t-u)^{\alpha(t)-1}(s-u)^{\alpha(s)-1}e^{2\omega u}du$$

$$= \frac{e^{-\omega(t-s)}}{\Gamma(\alpha(t))\Gamma(\alpha(s))}\int_0^\infty u^{\alpha(s)-1}(u+t-s)^{\alpha(t)-1}e^{-2\omega u}du$$

$$= \frac{e^{-\omega(t-s)}(t-s)^{\alpha(s)+\alpha(t)-1}}{\Gamma(\alpha(t))}\Psi\left(\alpha(s), \alpha(s)+\alpha(t), 2\omega(t-s)\right), \tag{23}$$

where $\Psi(\alpha, y; z)$ is the confluent hypergeometric function. In contrast to the Weyl fractional Ornstein-Uhlenbeck process, the multifractional process is in general not stationary.

For MOU process of RL type, its covariance for $s < t$ is

$$E\left(Y_{\alpha(t)}^{RL}(t)Y_{\alpha(s)}^{RL}(s)\right) = \frac{e^{-\omega(t+s)}}{\Gamma(\alpha(t))\Gamma(\alpha(s))}\int_0^s (t-u)^{\alpha(t)-1}(s-u)^{\alpha(s)-1}e^{2\omega u}du$$

$$= \frac{e^{-\omega(t+s)}s^{\alpha(s)}t^{\alpha(t)-1}}{\Gamma(\alpha(t))\Gamma(\alpha(s))}\int_0^1 (1-u)^{\alpha(s)-1}\left(1-\frac{s}{t}u\right)^{\alpha(t)-1}e^{2\omega us}du$$

$$= \frac{e^{-\omega(t+s)}s^{\alpha(s)}t^{\alpha(t)-1}}{\Gamma(\alpha(s)+1)\Gamma(\alpha(s))}\Phi_1\left(1, 1-\alpha(t), 1+\alpha(s), s/t, 2\omega(s)\right). \tag{24}$$

The local properties of these two types of MOU processes are similar to that of the corresponding MBM. With probability one, both the functions $Y_\alpha^W(t)$ and

$Y_\alpha^{RL}(t)$ have Hölder exponent $\alpha(t_\circ) - 1/2$ at the point $t_\circ$; and the Hausdorff dimension of the two processes is $5/2 - \alpha(t_\circ)$.[49] In addition, MOU processes of Weyl and RL-type are locally asymptotically self-similar, their tangent process at a point $t_\circ$ is the FBM indexed by parameter $\alpha(t_\circ) - 1/2$. In contrast to MBM, MOU processes are SRD, that is they are short memory processes.

The remark concerning the multifractality of the multifractional Brownian motion applies to the multifractional Ornstein-Uhlenbeck process. That is, the multifractional process is truly multifractal if the Hölder exponent is a random function, otherwise it is a multiscaling process. However, there are many phenomena that are multiscaling instead of multifractal.

5. Fractional and Multifractional Riesz-Bessel Motion

Fractional Riesz-Bessel motion (FRBM) was first introduced by Anh et al. as fractional Riesz-Bessel random field.[43] In one dimension, it is a Gaussian process parametrized by two indices which characterize separately two distinct properties — self-similarity and intermittency. The latter property corresponds to features such as sharp peaks or random bursts, and properties of processes that can be described by high skewed probability distributions with very slowly decaying tails. Thus FRBM has an advantage over FBM, which is unable to describe intermittency. In addition, for certain ranges of the two parameters, FRBM has a semimartingale representation.[44]

FRBM is closely related to Riesz and Bessel potentials. In the one dimension case, FRBM can be regarded as the solution of the following fractional stochastic differential equation:

$$D_t^{\gamma/2}(D_t + \omega)^{\alpha/2} V_{\alpha,\gamma} = \eta(t), \qquad\qquad \alpha \geq 0,\ 0 \leq \gamma < 1, \qquad (25)$$

where $D_t^{\gamma/2}$ is the Riesz derivative defined by

$$D_t^{\gamma/2} f(t) = F^{-1}\Big(|k|^\gamma \hat{f}(k)\Big), \qquad\qquad (26)$$

where F denotes Fourier transform, $\hat{f} = F(f)$. Formally, the solution of (25) is given by

$$V_{\alpha,\gamma}(t) = \frac{1}{2\pi} \int_{\mathbb{R}} \frac{e^{ikt}}{|k|^\gamma (\omega^2 + k^2)^{\alpha/2}} \eta(t) dt. \qquad\qquad (27)$$

(27) is to be regarded as a generalized random process.

Note that $V_{\alpha,\gamma}(t)$ can be defined as an ordinary stochastic process if $0 \leq \gamma < 1/2$, and $\alpha + \gamma > 1/2$. In the limit $\gamma = 0$, $V_{\alpha,\gamma}(t)$ becomes FOU process of Weyl type which is SRD. On the other hand, if $\alpha = 0$, (27) becomes the generalized spectral density associated with FBM, a long memory process. In general, $V_{\alpha,\gamma}(t)$ is LRD when $\gamma \neq 0$. Thus, FRBM allows interpolation between long and short memory processes.

The spectral density of $V_{\alpha,\gamma}(t)$ is

$$S(k) = \frac{1}{(2\pi)|k|^{2\gamma}(\omega^2 + k^2)^\alpha}. \tag{28}$$

The covariance of FRBM can be calculated as the inverse Fourier transform of the spectral density (28)

$$C_{\alpha,\gamma}(x) = \frac{\omega^{1-2\alpha-2\gamma}\Gamma\left(\frac{1}{2}-\gamma\right)\Gamma\left(\alpha+\gamma-\frac{1}{2}\right)}{2\pi\Gamma(\alpha)}\,_1F_2\left(\frac{1}{2}-\gamma;\frac{3}{2}-\alpha-\gamma,\frac{1}{2};\left[\frac{\omega|x|}{2}\right]^2\right)$$

$$+ \frac{|x|^{2\alpha+2\gamma-1}\Gamma\left(\frac{1}{2}-\alpha-\gamma\right)}{2^{2\alpha+2\gamma}\sqrt{\pi}\Gamma(\alpha+\gamma)}\,_1F_2\left(\alpha;\alpha+\gamma,\alpha+\gamma+\frac{1}{2};\left[\frac{\omega|x|}{2}\right]^2\right). \tag{29}$$

Note that when $\gamma = 0$, (29) becomes

$$C_{\alpha,0}(x) = \frac{2^{1/2-\alpha}}{\sqrt{\pi}\Gamma(\alpha)}\left(\frac{|x|}{\omega}\right)^{\alpha-1/2}K_{\alpha-1/2}(\omega|x|) \tag{30}$$

which is the covariance of the fractional Bessel process.[72] When $\alpha = 1$, (30) becomes the two-point Schwinger function of the one-dimensional Euclidean scalar massive field.

Additional properties of FRBM are discussed elsewhere.[43,44,51] Generalization of FRBM to multifractional RBM (MRBM) can again be carried out by replacing α and γ by $\alpha(t)$ and $\gamma(t)$ respectively in (27). The resulting MRBM $V_{\alpha(t),\gamma(t)}(t)$ is a Gaussian process which has many properties similar to MBM. For example, MRBM is locally asymptotically self-similar, its tangent process at a point t_o is a standard FBM indexed by $\alpha(t_o) + \gamma(t_o) - 1/2$. Note that this is an example of the general result of Falconer[73] that under certain conditions, the tangent process of a Gaussian process is FBM up to a multiplicative deterministic function of time. Another local property is that the Hausdorff dimension at a point t_o of the graph of FRBM is with probability one equal to $5/2 - \alpha(t_o) - \gamma(t_o)$.

Finally, we consider the LRD and SRD properties of MRBM. In the general case where $\alpha(t)$ and $\gamma(t)$ are not constants, we can show the following:[51] (a) If $\gamma(t) = 0$ and there exists a constant M so that $n/2 < \alpha(t) \leq M$ then the MRBM of variable order $V_{\alpha(t),0}(t)$ is SRD. (b) If there exist constants $L_1 \in (0, n/2)$ and $L_2 > n/2$, $M_1 \in (L_1, n/2)$, $M_2 \geq L_2$ so that $L_1 \leq \gamma(t) \leq M_1$ and $L_2 \leq \alpha(t) + \gamma(t) \leq M_2$, then MRBM $V_{\alpha(t),\gamma(t)}(t)$ is LRD.

FRBM and MRBM can be used to model systems that exhibit both long-range dependence and intermittency, for example, in financial time series, air pollution, rainfall data, porosity in heterogenous aquifer, turbulence, etc.[43,44,74–76]

6. Generalized Cauchy Process

The stationary Gaussian process defined by the following generalized Cauchy (GC) covariance parametrized by two indices

$$C_{\alpha,\beta}(t) = \left\langle U_{\alpha,\beta}(s)U_{\alpha,\beta}(t+s)\right\rangle = \left(1+|t|^\alpha\right)^{-\beta}, \quad t \in \mathbb{R},\ 0 < \alpha \leq 1,\ \beta > 0, \tag{31}$$

is known as generalized Cauchy process.[46] When $\alpha = 2$, $\beta = 1$ one gets the usual Cauchy process. This process was first introduced by Gneiting and Schlather.[45] It has a nice and useful property which allows separate characterization of fractal dimension and LRD by two different parameters.

It is well-known that a stationary process cannot be self-similar. $U_{\alpha,\beta}(t)$ satisfies a weaker self-similar property known as local self-similarity.[77,78] A Gaussian stationary process is locally self-similar of order κ if its covariance $C(t)$ satisfies for $t \to 0$,

$$C(t) = 1 - \beta|t|^{\kappa}\left[1 + O\big(|t|^{\nu}\big)\right], \qquad \nu > 0. \tag{32}$$

A more intuitive alternative definition is the following. A Gaussian process $U(t)$ is said to be locally self-similar of index κ if

$$U_{\alpha,\beta}(s) - U_{\alpha,\beta}(rt) = r^{\kappa}\left[U_{\alpha,\beta}(s) - U_{\alpha,\beta}(t)\right], \qquad \text{as } |t - s| \to 0, \tag{33}$$

where the equality is in the sense of finite joint distributions. The above two definitions and also the locally asymptotically self-similarity defined by (14) are all equivalent.[46] It is straightforward to show that the tangent process at a point t_{o} is FBM indexed by α. In other words, GC process behaves locally like a FBM. The fractal dimension of the graph of a locally self-similar process of order α is $5/2 - \alpha$.

GC process is LRD for $0 < \alpha\beta \leq 1$ and is SRD if $\alpha\beta > 1$. The large time lag behaviour of the covariance (31) is given by the hyperbolically decaying covariance $C(t) \sim |t|^{-\alpha\beta}$, $t \to \infty$ which is characteristic of LRD. If the covariance is re-expressed as $\big(1 + |t|^{\alpha}\big)^{-\zeta/\alpha}$ then the parameters α and ζ, respectively, provide separate characterization of fractal dimension and LRD.

It is interesting to point out that the covariance of GC process has the same functional form as the characteristic function of generalized Linnik distribution[79] and spectral density of the generalized Whittle-Matérn process.[72] There are also laws in physics which have this same analytic form. One example is the Havriliak-Negami relaxation law in the non-Debye relaxation theory.[46] Thus, all of these quantities should have the same analytic and asymptotic properties, and results obtained in any one of them are of relevance to the other.

Applications of GC process can be found in geostatistics, telecommunication and climate modelling.[46,80,81] Extension to GC field[82] is particularly useful for geological modeling. Generalization of GC process to multifractional GC process so far has not been carried out. However, it is expected such a generalization would be similar to MRBM indexed by two variable parameters.

7. Concluding Remarks

From the brief discussion given above, one notes that many of the fractional and multifractional Gaussian processes have similar local properties, in particular the local self-similarity (or having FBM as the tangent process at a point). The LRD (or SRD) character is carried over from the fractional process to the corresponding multifractional process. Some related processes such as step FBM[83] and mixed FBM[40] are not included. The step FBM can be regarded as a special case of MBM, with $H(t)$ a piecewise linear function. Such a multiscale process can be used to model anomalous transport phenomena such as single-file diffusion.[84] Mixed FBM is a linear combination of two or more independent FBM, and it can be used to model retarding anomalous diffusion,[85] financial time series,[31, 40] telecommunication,[86] etc. As far as applications of fractional and multifractional stochastic processes are concerned, it is possible to select from a variety of processes one that provides the best description of the system under study.

Finally, we remark that path integral formulation of fractional stochastic processes has recently attracted considerable interest from physicists as well as mathematicians.[87–90] In view of the fact that several candidate theories of quantum gravity[91–94] share the idea that spacetime is multifractal, one would expect path integral formulation of fractional and multifractional stochastic processes may play an important role in physics, just like the case in Brownian motion.

Acknowledgments

S. C. Lim would like to thank the organizers of this workshop, Chris and Victoria, for the financial support and their hospitality during his stay in Jagna.

References

1. K. B. Oldham and J. Spanier, *The Fractional Calculus: Theory and Application of Differentiation and Integration to Arbitrary Order* (London: Academic Press, 1974).
2. K. S. Miller and B. Ross, *An Introduction to the Fractional Calculus and Fractional Differential Equations* (New York: Wiley, 1993).
3. M. D. Ortigueira, *Fractional Calculus for Scientists and Engineers* (Springer, New York, 2011).
4. R. Herrmann, *Fractional Calculus: An Introduction for Physicists*, 2nd edn. (World Scientific, 2013).
5. R. Nigmatullin, *Theor. Math. Phys.* **90**, 242 (1992).
6. R. S. Rutman, *Theor. Math. Phys.* **105**, 1509 (1995).
7. F. B. Tatom, *Fractals* **3**, 217 (1995).
8. M. Moshrefi-Torbati and J. K. Hammond, *J. Franklin Inst. B* **335**, 1077-1086 (1998).
9. I. Podlubny, *J. Fract. Calc. Appl. Anal.* **5**, 357 (2002).
10. J. A. T. Machado, *J. Fract. Calc. Appl. Anal.* **6**, 73 (2003).
11. A. A. Stanislavsky, *Theor. Math. Phys.* **138**, 418 (2004).
12. S. G. Samko, A. A. Kilbas and O. I. Marichev, *Fractional Integrals and Derivatives: Theory and Applications* (New York: Gordon & Breach, 1993).
13. I. Podlubny, *Fractional Differential Equations* (San Diego: Academic Press, 1999).
14. A. A. Kilbas, H. M. Srivastava and J. J. Trujillo, *Theory and Applications of Fractional Differential Equations* (Elsevier Science & Technology, Amsterdam, 2006).
15. K. Diethelm, *The Analysis of Fractional Differential Equations* (Springer, New York, 2010).
16. R. Metzler and J. Klafter, *Physics Reports* **339**, 1 (2000).

17. R. Hilfer (ed.), *Applications of Fractional Calculus in Physics* (Singapore: World Scientific, 2000).
18. B. J. West, M. Bologna and P. Grigolini, *Physics of Fractal Operators* (New York: Springer, 2003).
19. G. M. Zaslavsky, *Hamiltonian Chaos and Fractional Dynamics* (Oxford: Oxford University, 2005).
20. R. Klages, G. Radons and I. M. Sokolov (eds.), *Anomalous Transport; Foundations and Applications.* (Wiley-VCH, New York,, 2008).
21. F. Mainardi, *Fractional Calculus and Waves in Linear Viscoelasticity: An Introduction to Mathematical Models* (Imperial College Press, London, 2010).
22. S. Das, *Functional Fractional Calculus for System Identification and Controls* (Springer, New York, 2011).
23. J. Klafter, S. C. Lim and R. Metzler (eds.), *Fractional Dynamics: Recent Advances* (World Scientific, Singapore, 2011).
24. V. E. Tarasov, *Fractional Dynamics: Applications of Fractional Calculus to Dynamics of Particles, Fields and Media* (Springer, New York, 2011).
25. K. Diethelm, D. Baleanu and E. Scalas, *Fractional Calculus: Models and Numerical Methods* (World Scientific, Singapore, 2012).
26. H. Sheng, Y. Q. Chen and T. S. Qiu, *Fractional Processes and Fractional-Order Signal Processing: Techniques and Applications* (Springer, New York, 2011).
27. M. M. Meerschaert and A. Sikorskii, *Stochastic Models for Fractional Calculus* (De Gruyter, Boston, 2012).
28. V. Uchaikin and R. Sibatov, *Fractional Kinetics in Solids: Anomalous Charge Transport in Semiconductors, Dielectrics and Nanosystems* (World Scientific, Singapore, 2012).
29. T. M. Atanackovic, S. Pilipovic, B. Stankovic and D. Zorica, *Fractional Calculus with Applications in Mechanics: Wave Propagation, Impact and Variational Principles* (Wiley-ISTE, New York, 2014).
30. F. Biagini, Y. Hu, B. Øksendal and T. Zhang, *Stochastic Calculus for Fractional Brownian Motion and Applications* (Springer, New York, 2008).
31. Y. Mishura, *Stochastic Calculus for Fractional Brownian Motion and Related Processes* (Springer, New York, 2008).
32. I. Nourdin, *Selected Aspects of Fractional Brownian Motion* (Springer, New York, 2012).
33. G. Samorodnitsky and M. S. Taqqu, *Stable Non-Gaussian Random Processes* (New York: Chapman and Hall, 1994).
34. T. Marquardt, *Bernoulli* **12**, 1099 (2006).
35. S. Cohen, A. Kuznetsov, A. E. Kyprianou and V. Rivero, *Lévy Matters II: Recent Progress in Theory and Applications: Fractional Lévy Fields, and Scale Functions* (Springer, New York, 2013).
36. P. Cheridito, H. Kawaguchi and M. Maejima, *Electron. J. Probab.* **8**, 1 (2003).
37. S. C. Lim and S. V. Muniandy, *J. Phys. A* **36**, 3961 (2003).
38. M. Magdziarz, *Physica A* **387**, 123 (2008).
39. F. Russo and C. A. Tudor, *Stochastic Process. Appl.* **116**, 830 (2006).
40. P. Cheridito, *Bernoulli* **7**, 913 (2001).
41. S. C. Lim, M. Li and L. P. Teo, *Phys. Lett. A* **372**, 6309 (2008).
42. S. C. Lim and L. P. Teo, *J. Phys. A: Math. Theor.* **42**, 065208 (34pp) (2009).
43. V. Anh, J. Angulo and M. Ruiz-Medina, *J. Statist. Plann. Inference* **80**, 95 (1999).
44. V. V. Anh, N. N. Leonenko and R. Mcvinish, *Fractals* **9**, 329 (2001).
45. T. Gneiting and M. Schlather, *SIAM Rev.* **46**, 269 (2004).

46. S. Lim and M. Li, *J. Phys. A: Math. Gen.* **39**, 2935 (2006).
47. R. Peltier and J. Lévy Véhel, *Multifractional Brownian Motion : Definition and Preliminary Results*, Rapport de recherche RR-2645, INRIA (1995),
48. A. Benassi, S. Jaffard and D. Roux, *Rev. Mat. Iber.* **13**, 19 (1997).
49. S. C. Lim and L. P. Teo, *J. Phys. A: Math. Gen.* **40**, 6035 (2007).
50. M. D. Ruiz-Medina, V. V. Anh and J. M. Angulo, *Stochastic Anal. Appl.* **22**, 775 (2004).
51. S. C. Lim and L. P. Teo, *J. Math. Phys.* **49**, 013509 (2008).
52. B. B. Mandelbrot and J. W. van Ness, *SIAM Rev.* **10**, 422 (1968).
53. J. A. Barnes and D. W. Allan, *Proc. IEEE* **54**, 170 (1966).
54. O. Sheluhin, S. Smolskiy and A. Osin, *Self-Similar Processes in Telecommunications* (John Wiley & Sons, Southern Gate, Chichester, 2007).
55. S. Rostek, *Option Pricing in Fractional Brownian Markets* (Springer, New York, 2009).
56. Y. Kobelev, L. Kobelev and Y. Klimontovich, *Phys. Dokl.* **48**, 264 (2003).
57. Y. Kobelev, L. Kobelev and Y. Klimontovich, *Phys. Dokl.* **48**, 285 (2003).
58. H. G. Sun, W. Chen and Y. Q. Chen, *Physica A* **388**, 4586 (2009).
59. S. Cohen, From self-similarity to local self-similarity: the estimation problem, in *Fractals*, eds. M. Dekking, J. Lévy-Véhel, E. Lutton and C. Tricot (Springer London, 1999), pp. 3–16.
60. S. C. Lim and S. V. Muniandy, *Phys. Lett. A* **266**, 140 (2000).
61. S. C. Lim, *J. Phys. A: Math. Gen.* **34**, 1301 (2001).
62. P. M. Krishna, V. M. Gadre and U. B. Desai, *Multifractal Based Network Traffic Modeling* (Springer New York, 2003).
63. H. Sheng, Y. Q. Chen and T. S. Qiu, *Fractional Processes and Fractional-Order Signal Processing: Techniques and Applications* (Springer, New York, 2012), ch. 6, pp. 149–160.
64. S. Gaci, J. Lévy-Véhel, C. Keylock and J. W. and. D. Schertzer (eds.), *Nonlinear Processes in Geophysics on Multifractional Brownian Motions in Geosciences* 2012.
65. A. Echelard, O. Barriére and J. Lévy-Véhel, Terrain modeling with multifractional brownian motion and self-regulating processes, in *Computer Vision and Graphics*, Lecture Notes in Computer Science Vol. 6374 (Springer Berlin Heidelberg, 2010), pp. 342–351.
66. S. Corlay, J. Lebovits and J. L. Véhel, *Math. Finance* **24**, 364 (2014).
67. S. C. Lim and S. V. Muniandy, *Phys. Rev. E* **66**, 021114 (2002).
68. T. Marguez-Lago, A. Leier and K. Burrage, *IET Syst Biol* **6**, 134 (2012).
69. A. Ayache and J. L. Véhel, *Stat. Inference Stoch. Process.* **3**, 7 (2000).
70. J. L. Véhel, *Nonlinear Process. Geophys.* **20**, 643 (2013).
71. S. C. Lim and C. H. Eab, *Phys. Lett. A* **335**, 87 (2006).
72. S. C. Lim and L. P. Teo, *J. Phys. A: Math. Theor.* **42**, 105202 (21pp) (2009).
73. K. J. Falconer, *J. Lond. Math. Soc.* **67**, 657 (2003).
74. J. Gao, V. V. Anh and C. Heyde, *Stochastic Process. Appl.* **99**, 295 (2002).
75. V. V. Anh, J. M. Angulo, M. D. Ruiz-Medina and Q. Tieng, *Environ. Model. Software* **13**, 233 (1998).
76. J. Gao, *J. Appl. Probab.* **41**, 467 (2004).
77. J. T. Kent and A. T. A. Wood, *J. R. Stat. Soc. B* **59**, 679 (1997).
78. A. J. Adler, *The Geometry of Random Fields* (New York: Wiley, 1981).
79. S. C. Lim and L. P. Teo, *J. Fourier Anal. Appl.* **16**, 715 (2010).
80. M. Li and S. C. Lim, *Physica A* **387**, 387, 2584 (2008).
81. M. Schlather, *Bernoulli* **16**, 780 (2010).
82. S. Lim and L. Teo, *Stochastic Process. Appl.* **119**, 1325 (2009).

83. A. Benassi, P. Bertrand, S. Cohen and J. Istas, *Stat. Inference Stoch. Process.* **3**, 101 (2000).
84. S. C. Lim and L. P. Teo, *J. Stat. Mech.* **2009**, p. P08015 (2009).
85. C. H. Eab and S. L. Lim, *J. Phys. A: Math. Theor.* **45**, 145001 (2012).
86. D. Filatova, Mixed fractional Brownian motion: some related questions for computer network traffic modelling, in *International Conference on Signal and Electronic Systems*, 2008, pp. 393–396.
87. H. S. Wio, *Path Integrals for Stochastic Processes: An Introduction* (Singapore: World Scientific, 2013), see also additional references quoted in the book.
88. H. Kleinert, *Europhys. Lett.* **100**, 10001 (2012).
89. D. Janakiraman and K. L. Sebastian, *Phys. Rev. E* **86**, 061105 (2012).
90. C. H. Eab and S. C. Lim, preprint arXiv:1405.0653 (2014).
91. L. Modesto, *Class. Quant. Grav.* **26**, 242002 (2009).
92. J. Ambjørn, A. Görlich, J. Jurkiewicz and R. Loll, *Phys. Lett. B* **690**, 420 (2010).
93. G. Calcagni, *Phys. Rev. Lett.* **104**, 251301 (2010).
94. G. Calcagni, *Journal of High Energy Physics* **2012:65** (2012).

7th Jagna International Workshop (2014)
International Journal of Modern Physics: Conference Series
Vol. 36 (2015) 1560002 (16 pages)
© The Author
DOI: 10.1142/S2010194515600022

World Scientific
www.worldscientific.com

Fractional Brownian motion in a nutshell

Georgiy Shevchenko

Department of Mechanics and Mathematics,
Taras Shevchenko National University of Kyiv
Volodymirska 60, 01601 Kyiv, Ukraine
zhora@univ.kiev.ua

Published 2 January 2015

This is an extended version of the lecture notes to a mini-course devoted to fractional Brownian motion and delivered to the participants of the 7th Jagna International Workshop.

Keywords: Fractional Brownian motion; Hurst parameter; Hölder continuity; consistent estimation; simulation.

1. Introduction

The fractional Brownian motion (fBm) is a popular model for both short-range dependent and long-range dependent phenomena in various fields, including physics, biology, hydrology, network research, financial mathematics, etc. There are many good sources devoted to the fBm, I will cite only few of them. For a good introductory text on the fBm, a reader may address recent Ivan Nourdin's lecture notes[1] or the dedicated chapter of the famous David Nualart's book.[2] More comprehensive guides are by Yuliya Mishura[3] and Francesca Biagini et al;[4] the former has stronger emphasis towards the pathwise integration, while the latter, towards the white noise approach. A review of Jean-François Coeurjolly[5] is an extensive guide to the use of statistical methods and simulation procedures for the fBm.

It is worth saying few words on the aim and the origin of this article. After I gave a mini-course devoted to the fBm at the 7th Jagna International Conference, the organizers approached me with a proposition to write lecture notes. Knowing that there are already so many sources devoted to the fBm, I was hesitant for the first time. But ultimately I decided to agree and wrote this article. Naturally, it would be impossible to cover all the aspects of the fBm in such a short exposition, and this was not my aim. My aim was rather to make a brief introduction to the fBm. Since most of the listeners of the course were not pure mathematicians, I tried to keep the text as accessible as possible, at the same time paying more attention at such practical issues as the simulation and identification of fBm.

The article is structured as follows. In Section 2, the fractional Brownian motion is defined, and its essential properties are studied. Section 3 is devoted to the continuity of fBm. In Section 4, several integral representations of fBm in terms of standard Wiener process are given. Section 5 discusses the statistical estimation issues for fBm. In Section 6, a simulation algorithm for fBm is presented.

2. Definition and Basic Properties

Definition 2.1. A *fractional Brownian motion* (fBm) is a centered Gaussian process $\{B_t^H, t \geq 0\}$ with the covariance function

$$\mathsf{E}\left[B_t^H B_s^H\right] = \frac{1}{2}\left(t^{2H} + s^{2H} - |t-s|^{2H}\right). \tag{1}$$

This process has a parameter $H \in (0,1)$, called the *Hurst parameter* or the *Hurst index*.

Remark 2.1. In order to specify the distribution of a Gaussian process, it is enough to specify its mean and covariance function, therefore, for each fixed value of the Hurst parameter H, the distribution of B^H is uniquely determined by the above definition. However, this definition does not guarantee the existence of fBm; to show that the fBm exists, one needs e.g. to check that the covariance function is non-negative definite. We will show the existence later, in Section 4, giving an explicit construction of fBm.

Observe that for $H = 1/2$, the covariance function is $\mathsf{E}\left[B_t^{1/2} B_s^{1/2}\right] = t \wedge s$, i.e. $B^{1/2} = W$, a standard Wiener process, or a Brownian motion. This justifies the name "fractional Brownian motion": B^H is a generalization of Brownian motion obtained by allowing the Hurst parameter to differ from $1/2$. Later we will uncover the meaning of the Hurst parameter.

Further we study several properties which can be deduced immediately from the definition. The following representation for the covariance of increments of fBm is easily obtained from (1):

$$\mathsf{E}\left[\left(B_{t_1}^H - B_{s_1}^H\right)\left(B_{t_2}^H - B_{s_2}^H\right)\right]$$
$$= \frac{1}{2}\left(|t_1 - s_2|^{2H} + |t_2 - s_1|^{2H} - |t_2 - t_1|^{2H} - - |s_2 - s_1|^{2H}\right). \tag{2}$$

Stationary increments. Take a fixed $t \geq 0$ and consider the process $Y_t = B_{t+s}^H - B_s^H$, $t \geq 0$. It follows from (2) that the covariance function of Y is the same as that of B^H. Since the both processes are centered Gaussian, the equality of covariance functions implies that Y has the same distribution as B^H. Thus, the incremental behavior of B^H at any point in the future is the same, for this reason

B^H is said to have stationary increments. Processes with stationary increments are good for modeling a time-homogeneous evolution of system.

Self-similarity. Now consider, for a fixed $a > 0$, the process $Z_t = B_{at}^H$, $t \geq 0$. It is clearly seen from (1) that Z has the same covariance, consequently, the same distribution as $a^H B^H$. This property is called H-self-similarity. It means the scale-invariance of the process: in each time interval the behavior is the same, if we choose the space scale properly.

It is an easy exercise to show that the fBm with Hurst parameter H is, up to a constant, the only H-self-similar Gaussian process with stationary increments.

Dependence of increments. Let us return to the formula (2) and study it in more detail. Assume that $s_1 < t_1 < s_2 < t_2$ so that the intervals $[s_1, t_1]$ and $[s_2, t_2]$ do not intersect. Then the left-hand side of (2) can be expressed as $((f(a_1) - f(a_2) - (f(b_1) - f(b_2))/2$, where $a_1 = t_2 - s_1$, $a_2 = t_2 - t_1$, $b_1 = s_2 - s_1$, $b_2 = s_2 - t_1$, $f(x) = x^{2H}$. Obviously, $a_1 - a_2 = b_2 - b_1 = t_1 - s_1$. Therefore,

$$\mathsf{E}\left[\left(B_{t_1}^H - B_{s_1}^H \right) \left(B_{t_2}^H - B_{s_2}^H \right) \right] < 0 \quad \text{for } H \in (0, 1/2)$$

in view of the concavity of f;

$$\mathsf{E}\left[\left(B_{t_1}^H - B_{s_1}^H \right) \left(B_{t_2}^H - B_{s_2}^H \right) \right] > 0 \quad \text{for } H \in (1/2, 1),$$

since f is convex in this case. Thus, for $H \in (0, 1/2)$, the fBm has the property of counterpersistence: if it was increasing in the past, it is more likely to decrease in the future, and vice versa. In contrast, for $H \in (1/2, 1)$, the fBm is persistent, it is more likely to keep trend than to break it. Moreover, for such H, the fBm has the property of long memory (long-range dependence).

Finally we mention that the fBm is neither a Markov process nor a semimartingale.

3. Continuity of Fractional Brownian Motion

There are several ways to establish the continuity of fBm. All of them are based on the formula

$$\mathsf{E}\left[\left(B_t^H - B_s^H \right)^2 \right] = |t - s|^{2H} \tag{3}$$

for the variogram of fBm, which follows from (2).

The first of the methods is probably the most popular way to prove that a process is continuous.

Theorem 3.1 (Kolmogorov–Chentsov continuity theorem). *Assume that for a stochastic process $\{X_t, t \geq 0\}$ there exist such $K > 0, p > 0, \beta > 0$ such that for all $t \geq 0, s \geq 0$*

$$\mathsf{E}\left[|X_t - X_s|^p \right] \leq K |t - s|^{1+\beta}.$$

Then the process X has a continuous modification, i.e. a process $\left\{ \widetilde{X}_t, t \geq 0 \right\}$ such that $\widetilde{X} \in C[0, \infty)$ and for all $t \geq 0$ $\Pr(X_t = \widetilde{X}_t) = 1$. Moreover, for any $\gamma \in (0, \beta/p)$

and $T > 0$ the process $\widetilde{X}$ is γ-Hölder continuous on $[0, T]$, i.e.

$$\sup_{0 \le s < t \le T} \frac{|X_t - X_s|}{(t-s)^\gamma} < \infty.$$

Corollary 3.1. *The fractional Brownian motion B^H has continuous modification. Moreover, for any $\gamma \in (0, H)$ this modification is γ-Hölder continuous on each finite interval.*

Proof. Since $B_t^H - B_s^H$ is centered Gaussian with variance $|t - s|^H$, we have $\mathsf{E}\left[\left| B_t^H - B_s^H \right|^p \right] = K_p |t - s|^{pH}$. Therefore, taking any $p > 1/H$, we get the existence of continuous modification. We also get the Hölder continuity of the modification with exponent $\gamma \in (0, H - 1/p)$. Choosing p sufficiently large, we arrive at the desired statement. $\qquad \square$

To avoid speaking about a continuous modification each time, in the rest of this article we will assume the continuity of fBm itself.

Another way to argue the Hölder continuity lies through a very powerful deterministic inequality.

Theorem 3.2 (Garsia–Rodemich–Rumsey inequality). *For any $p > 0$ and $\theta > 1/p$ there exists a constant $K_{p,\theta}$ such that for any $f \in C[0, T]$*

$$\sup_{0 \le s < t \le T} \frac{|f(t) - f(s)|}{(t-s)^{\theta - 1/p}} \le C_{p,\theta} \left(\int_0^T \int_0^T \frac{|f(x) - f(y)|^p}{|x - y|^{\theta p + 1}} \, dx \, dy \right)^{1/p}.$$

Remark 3.1. One of the most widely used techniques in calculus is the estimation of integral by the supremum of integrand times measure of integration set, e.g. $\left| \int_a^b f(x) dx \right| \le \sup_{x \in [a,b]} |f(x)| (b - a)$. However, obviously, one cannot reverse this inequality and estimate the integrand by the value of integral (although the temptation is great sometimes). Now we see why the Garsia–Rodemich–Rumsey (GRR) inequality is a very striking fact (at least at first glance): it is a valid example of such reverse statement.

The continuity assumption in the GRR inequality is essential. It is easy to see that for $f = \mathbf{1}_{[0, T/2]}$ the right-hand side of the inequality is finite, while the left-hand side is infinite. So in order to show the Hölder continuity of fBm using the GRR inequality, we should first establish usual continuity with the help of some other methods (and we have already done that). The advantage of the GRR inequality is that in contast to the Kolmogorov–Chentsov theorem it allows to estimate the Hölder norm of a process.

Alternative proof of the second part of Corollary 3.1. We remind that we assume B^H itself to be continuous. Take some $\theta < H$ and $p > 1/H$ and write, as before, $\mathsf{E}\left[\left|B_t^H - B_s^H\right|^p\right] = K_p \left|t - s\right|^{pH}$. Denote

$$\zeta = \sup_{0 \leq s < t \leq T} \frac{\left|B_t^H - B_s^H\right|}{(t-s)^{\theta - 1/p}}.$$

Raising the GRR inequality to the power p and taking expectations, we get

$$\mathsf{E}\left[\zeta^p\right] \leq K_{p,\theta}^p \int_0^T \int_0^T \frac{\mathsf{E}\left[\left|B_x^H - B_y^H\right|^p\right]}{\left|x - y\right|^{\theta p + 1}} \, dx \, dy$$

$$= K_{p,\theta}^p K_p \int_0^T \int_0^T \left|x - y\right|^{p(H-\theta)-1} \, dx \, dy < \infty.$$

It follows that $\zeta < \infty$ a.s. By changing, if necessary, the fBm B^H on an event of zero probability, we get the desired Hölder continuity. □

Finally, we mention that by using specialized facts about regularity of Gaussian processes, it is possible to show that the exact modulus of continuity of fBm is $\omega(\delta) = \delta^H \left|\log \delta\right|^{1/2}$. Consequently, it is only Hölder continuous of order up to H, but not H-Hölder continuous (although quite close to be).

Let us now summarize what we know about the Hurst parameter H. We already knew that, depending on whether $H \in (0, 1/2)$ or $H \in (1/2, 1)$, the increments of fBm are either negatively correlated or positively correlated. It is also easy to see that the correlation increases with H. In other words, the fBm becomes more and more persistent when H increases (ultimately for $H = 1$ it becomes a linear function: $B_t^1 = \xi t$, where ξ is standard Gaussian).

On the other hand, it follows from the above discussion that the Hurst parameter H dictates the regularity of fBm: the larger H is, the smoother fBm becomes. Now it is probably the most suitable moment to give some pictures of fBm, which illustrate perfectly the dependence of fBm on H.

4. Integral Representations of Fractional Brownian Motion

Further we will study representations of fractional Brownian motion in terms of a standard Wiener process. I expect the reader to be aware of Itô stochastic calculus, nevertheless, it is worth to give concise information on the objects we need.

Let $\{W_t, t \geq \mathbb{R}\}$ be a standard Wiener process on $\mathbb{R}$, i.e. $\{W_t, t \geq 0\}$ and $\{W_{-t}, t \geq 0\}$ are independent standard Wiener processes on $[0, \infty)$.

For functions $f \in L^2(\mathbb{R})$ the integral $I(f) = \int_{\mathbb{R}} f(x) dW(x)$ with respect to W (the Wiener integral) is constructed as follows. For a step function

$$h(x) = \sum_{k=1}^n a_k \mathbf{1}_{[s_k, t_k]}(x),$$

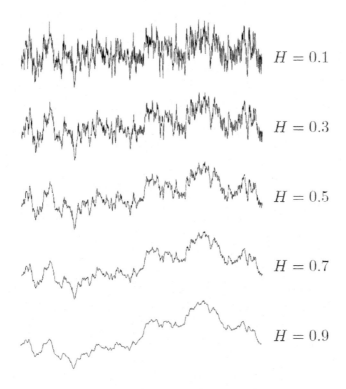

Fig. 1.   Paths of fBm for different values of H.

define

$$I(h) = \int_{\mathbb{R}} h(x)dW(x) = \sum_{k=1}^{n} a_k \left(W_{t_k} - W_{s_k} \right).$$

It is easily checked that I is linear and isometric, consequently, it can be extended from the set of step functions to $L^2(\mathbb{R})$. This extension, naturally, is an isometry too. We summarize below its basic properties.

1. linearity: for $\alpha, \beta \in \mathbb{R}$, $f, g \in L^2(\mathbb{R})$

$$I(\alpha f + \beta g) = \alpha I(f) + \beta I(g);$$

2. mean zero: $\mathsf{E}\left[I(f)\right] = 0$;
3. isometry: $\mathsf{E}\left[I(f)^2\right] = \int_{\mathbb{R}} f(x)^2 dx$, moreover, for $f, g \in L^2(\mathbb{R})$

$$\mathsf{E}\left[I(f)I(g)\right] = \int_{\mathbb{R}} f(x)g(x)dx.$$

4. for $f_1, \ldots, f_n \in L^2(\mathbb{R})$ the random variables $I(f_1), \ldots, I(f_n)$ are jointly Gaussian.

Next we consider representations of the form

$$B_t^H = I(k_t) = \int_{\mathbb{R}} k_t(x)dW(x),$$

where for each $t \geq 0$ $k_t \in L^2(\mathbb{R})$ is some deterministic kernel (not necessarily supported by the whole real line). Due to the properties of Wiener integral, the process given by such representation is a centered Gaussian process. So in order to argue that such representation defines an fBm, it is enough to show that it has the same covariance. The following simple statement may also be of use: a process has covariance given by (1) iff its variogram is given by (3).

The *Mandelbrot–Van Ness* representation, or the moving average representation of fBm is defined in the following proposition. It also can be used as a proof of existence of fBm.

Theorem 4.1. *Let for $H \in (0,1)$*

$$k_t^{MA}(x) = K_H^{MA}\left((t-x)_+^{H-1/2}\mathbf{1}_{(-\infty,0)}(x) - (-x)_+^{H-1/2}\right),$$

where

$$
\begin{aligned}
K_H^{MA} &= \left(\frac{1}{2H} + \int_0^\infty \left((x+1)^{H-1/2} - x^{H-1/2}\right)^2 dx\right)^{-1/2} \\
&= \frac{(\Gamma(2H+1)\sin \pi H)^{1/2}}{\Gamma(H+1/2)}.
\end{aligned}
$$

Then the process $X_t = I(k_t^{MA})$ is an fBm with Hurst parameter H.

Proof. As it was already mentioned above, in order to prove the statement, it suffices to show that for any $t, s \geq 0$ $\mathsf{E}\left[(X_t - X_s)^2\right] = |t - s|^{2H}$.

Write, denoting $\mu = H - 1/2$,

$$
\begin{aligned}
\mathsf{E}\left[(X_t - X_s)^2\right] &= (K_H^{MA})^2 \int_{\mathbb{R}} \left((t-x)_+^\mu - (s-x)_+^\mu\right)^2 dx \\
&= (K_H^{MA})^2 (t-s)^{2H} \int_{\mathbb{R}} \left((x+1)_+^\mu - (x)_+^\mu\right)^2 dx \\
&= (K_H^{MA})^2 (t-s)^2 H \left(\int_{-1}^0 (x+1)^{2H-1} dx + \int_0^\infty \left((x+1)^\mu - x^\mu\right)^2 dx\right) \\
&= (t-s)^{2H},
\end{aligned}
$$

as required. We will omit the proof of the second formula for K_H^{MA}, an interested reader may refer to Appendix in Ref. 3. $\qquad\square$

Let us now turn to the harmonizable representation of fBm.

Theorem 4.2. *Let for $H \in (0,1)$*

$$k_t^{Ha}(x) = K_H^{Ha} |x|^{-H-1/2} \begin{cases} \sin tx, & x \geq 0, \\ 1 - \cos tx, & x < 0, \end{cases}$$

where

$$K_H^{Ha} = \left(2\int_0^\infty \frac{1-\cos x}{x^{2H+1}dx}\right)^{-1/2} = \frac{(2\Gamma(2H+1)\sin\pi H)^{1/2}}{\pi}.$$

Then the process $X_t = I(k_t^{Ha})$ is an fBm with Hurst parameter H.

Proof. As in the previous proof, write

$$\mathsf{E}\left[(X_t - X_s)^2\right] = (K_H^{Ha})^2\left[\int_0^\infty \frac{(\sin tx - \sin sx)^2}{x^{2H+1}}dx + \int_{-\infty}^0 \frac{(\cos tx - \cos sx)^2}{(-x)^{2H+1}}dx\right]$$

$$= (K_H^{Ha})^2\int_0^\infty \frac{2 - 2\cos(t-s)x}{x^{2H+1}}dx$$

$$= 2(K_H^{Ha})^2(t-s)^{2H}\int_0^\infty \frac{1-\cos z}{z^{2H+1}}dx = (t-s)^{2H}.$$

Again, we do not prove the second formula for K_H^{Ha}. $\qquad\square$

The third representation we consider, the so-called Volterra type representation, is a bit more involved than the former two, but its advantage is that the kernel in this representation has compact support.

Theorem 4.3. *Let for $H \in (1/2, 1)$*

$$k_t^V(x) = K_H^V x^{1/2-H}\int_x^t s^{H-1/2}(s-x)^{H-3/2}ds\,\mathbf{1}_{[0,t]}(x),$$

where

$$K_H^V = \left(\frac{H(2H-1)}{B(2-2H, H-1/2)}\right)^{1/2} = K_H^{MA};$$

for $H \in (0, 1/2)$,

$$k_t^V(x) = K_H^V x^{1/2-H}\left(t^{H-1/2}(t-x)^{H-1/2}\right.$$

$$\left. - (H-1/2)x^{1/2-H}\int_x^t s^{H-3/2}(s-x)^{H-1/2}ds\right)\mathbf{1}_{[0,t]}(x),$$

where

$$K_H^V = \left(\frac{2H}{(1-2H)B(1-2H, H+1/2)}\right)^{1/2}.$$

Then $X_t = I(k_t^V)$ is an fBm with Hurst parameter H.

Proof. We will consider only the case $H \in (1/2, 1)$, the other case being somewhat similar but a lot more tricky.

Denote $\mu = H - 1/2$ and write for $t, s \geq 0$

$$\mathsf{E}[X_t X_s] = (K_H^V)^2 \int_0^{t \wedge s} x^{-2\mu} \int_x^t u^\mu (u-x)^{\mu-1} du \int_x^s v^\mu (v-x)^{\mu-1} dv \, dx$$

$$= (K_H^V)^2 \int_0^t \int_0^s u^\mu v^\mu \int_0^{u \wedge v} x^{-2\mu}(u-x)^{\mu-1}(v-x)^{\mu-1} dx \, dv \, du.$$

For $u \leq v$, make the change of variable $z = \frac{1-x/u}{1-x/v}$ in the inner integral so that $x = \frac{uv(1-z)}{v-zu}$, $u - x = \frac{uz(v-u)}{v-zu}$, $v - x = \frac{v(v-u)}{v-zu}$, $dx = -\frac{uv(v-u)}{(v-zu)^2}$ to obtain

$$\int_0^u x^{-2\mu}(u-x)^{\mu-1}(v-x)^{\mu-1} dx$$

$$= \int_0^1 \frac{(v-zu)^{2\mu}}{(uv)^{2\mu}(1-z)^{2\mu}} \frac{(uz)^{\mu-1}(v-u)^{\mu-1}}{(v-zu)^{\mu-1}} \frac{v^{\mu-1}(v-u)^{\mu-1}}{(v-zu)^{\mu-1}} \frac{uv(v-u)}{(v-zu)^2} dz$$

$$= u^{-\mu} v^{-\mu} (v-u)^{2\mu-1} \int_0^1 z^{\mu-1}(1-z)^{-2\mu} dz$$

$$= u^{-\mu} v^{-\mu} (v-u)^{2H-2} \mathrm{B}(2-2H, H-1/2),$$

and a similar formula is valid for $v \leq u$. Substituting this into the above expression for $\mathsf{E}[X_t X_s]$, we arrive at

$$\mathsf{E}[X_t X_s] = H(2H-1) \int_0^t \int_0^s |v-u|^{2H-2} du = \frac{1}{2}\left(t^{2H} + s^{2H} - |t-s|^{2H}\right),$$

as required. $\qquad\qquad\square$

5. Identification of Hurst Parameter

In order to use a stochastic process as a model in practice, one needs a good statistical machinery. There are many statistical tools available for models based on the fBm, and this article is too short to cover them all. The most important statistical question is about the Hurst parameter, which governs all essential properties of fBm.

Consider the following statistical problem: to estimate the Hurst parameter H based on the observations $B_1^H, B_2^H, \ldots, B_N^H$ of fBm, where N is large. There are several approaches to this problem. We will study here only an approach based on discrete variations of fBm, further methods can be found in.[5]

First we need to destroy the dependence by applying a suitable filter. Specifically, a filter of order r is a polynomial $a(x) = \sum_{k=0}^q a_k x^k$ such that $a(1) = a'(1) = \cdots = a^{(r-1)}(1) = 0$, $a^{(r)}(1) \neq 0$ (equivalently, 1 is the root of polynomial a of multiplicity

r). The filtered observations are defined as

$$B_n^a = \sum_{k=0}^{q} a_k B_{n+k}^H, \quad n = 1, 2, \ldots, N - q.$$

Popular filters are Increments 1 with $a(x) = x - 1$, Daubechies 4 with $a(x) = \frac{1}{4}(x-1)(x^2(1-\sqrt{3}) - 2x)$, Increments 2 with $a(x) = (x-1)^2$. The first two filters are of order 1, the third, of order 2. As it was mentioned, the main aim of filtering is to reduce dependence of the data. Indeed, for a filter a of order $r \geq 1$ consider the covariance

$$\mathsf{E}\left[B_n^a B_m^a \right] = \sum_{k=0}^{q} \sum_{j=0}^{q} a_k a_j \mathsf{E}\left[B_{n+k}^H B_{n+k}^H \right]$$

$$= \frac{1}{2} \sum_{k=0}^{q} \sum_{j=0}^{q} a_k a_j \left((n+k)^{2H} + (m+j)^{2H} - |m+k-n-j|^{2H} \right)$$

$$= \frac{1}{2} \left(\sum_{k=0}^{q} a_k (n+k)^{2H} \sum_{j=0}^{q} a_j + \sum_{j=0}^{q} a_j (m+j)^{2H} \sum_{k=0}^{q} a_k \right.$$

$$\left. - \sum_{k=0}^{q} \sum_{j=0}^{q} a_k a_j |m+k-n-j|^{2H} \right)$$

$$= -\frac{1}{2} \sum_{k=0}^{q} \sum_{j=0}^{q} a_k a_j |m-n+k-j|^{2H} =: \rho_H^a(m-n),$$

where we have used that $\sum_{k=0}^{q} a_k = a(1) = 0$. Consequently, the filtered data $B_1^a, \ldots, B_{N-q}^a$ is a stationary process. Moreover, since $(x-1)^r \mid a(x)$, in the expression for ρ_H^a one takes the finite difference of the function x^{2H} $2r$ times: r times with respect to n and r times with respect to m. It follows that $\rho_H^a(n) \sim K_{H,a} n^{2(H-r)}$, thus the covariance indeed decays faster for large r.

To define an estimator for the Hurst coefficient, for $m \geq 1$ consider the dilated filter $a^m(x) := a(x^m) = \sum_{k=0}^{q} a_k x^{km}$. It is obvious that $\rho_H^{a^m}(0) = m^{2H} \rho_H^a(0)$, equivalently,

$$\log \rho_H^{a^m}(0) = 2H \log m + \rho_H^a(0). \tag{4}$$

Thus, an estimator for H may be obtained by taking a linear regression of estimators for $\log \rho_H^{a^m}(0)$ on $\log m$. To estimate $\rho_H^{a^m}(0)$ consistently, one can use the empiric moments.

Theorem 5.1. *The empiric variance*

$$V_N^{a^m} = \frac{1}{N - mq} \sum_{k=1}^{N-mq} \left(B_k^{a^m} \right)^2$$

is a strongly consistent estimator of $r_H^{a^m}(0)$, *i.e.* $V_N^{a^m} \to r_H^{a^m}(0)$ *a.s. as* $N \to \infty$.

Proof. Since the sequence $\left\{B_k^{a^m}, k \geq 1\right\}$ is stationary, the result follows immediately from the ergodic theorem. □

Corollary 5.1. *Let a set $M \subset \mathbb{N}$ contain at least two elements, and $\widehat{k}_N^{a,M}$ be the coefficient of linear regression of $\left\{\log V_N^{a^m}, m \in M\right\}$ on $\{\log m, m \in M\}$. Then the statistic $\widehat{H}_N^{a,M} = \widehat{k}_N^{a,M}/2$ is a strongly consistent estimator of H.*

Proof. Follows directly from Theorem 5.1 and equation 4. □

Remark 5.1. Evidently, the same procedure can be used to estimate the Hurst parameter from observations $cB_1^H, cB_2^H, \dots, cB_N^H$ of fBm multiplied by an unknown scale coefficient c. This will not cause any problem, as in (4) we would have an extra term $\log c$, which does not influence the estimation procedure. Moreover, thanks to the self-similarity property, the estimation procedure will not change if the scaled fBm is observed not at the positive integer points, but at the points of some other equidistant grid, i.e. if one observes the values $cB_\Delta^H, cB_{2\Delta}^H, \dots, cB_{N\Delta}^H$. It is even possible to take $\Delta = T/N$ so that we observe the values on some fixed interval. However, one needs a different *strong* consistency proof, as in this case the ergodic theorem gives only the convergence in probability.

The simplest example of the regression set M in Corollary 5.1 is $M = \{1, 2\}$, and the simplest example of the filter is Increments 1, $d(x) = x - 1$. We get the following standard strongly consistent estimator of H:

$$\widehat{H}_k = \frac{1}{2} = \frac{1}{2 \log 2}(\log V_N^{d^2} - \log V_N^d) = \frac{1}{2} \log_2 \frac{V_N^{d^2}}{V_N^d},$$

where

$$V_N^d = \frac{1}{N-1} \sum_{k=1}^{N-1} \left(B_{k+1}^H - B_k^H\right)^2, \quad V_N^{d^2} = \frac{1}{N-2} \sum_{k=1}^{N-1} \left(B_{k+2}^H - B_k^H\right)^2.$$

Let us now turn to the asymptotic normality of the coefficients. We start by formulating a rather general statement.

Let $\xi_1, \xi_2, \dots$ be a stationary sequence of standard Gaussian variables with covariance $\rho(n) = \mathsf{E}\left[\xi_1 \xi_{n+1}\right]$, and $g \colon \mathbb{R} \to \mathbb{R}$ be a function such that $\mathsf{E}\left[g(\xi_1)\right] = 0$, $\mathsf{E}\left[g(\xi_1)^2\right] < \infty$. The latter assumption means that $g \in L^2(\mathbb{R}, \gamma)$, where γ is the standard Gaussian measure on $\mathbb{R}$. Consequently, g can be expanded in a series $g(x) = \sum_{k=0}^{\infty} g_k H_k(x)$ with respect to a system $\{H_k, k \geq 0\}$ of orthogonal polynomials for the measure γ, which are Hermite polynomials. We have $g_0 = \mathsf{E}\left[g(\xi_1)\right] = 0$. The smallest number p such that $g_p \neq 0$ is called the Hermite rank of g.

The following theorem describes the limit behavior of the cumulative sums $S_N = \sum_{k=1}^{N} g(\xi_k)$.

Theorem 5.2 (Breuer–Major). *Assume that $\sum_{n=1}^{\infty} |\rho(n)|^p < \infty$. Then one has the following convergence in finite-dimensional distributions:*

$$\left\{ \frac{1}{\sqrt{N}} S_{[Nt]}, t \geq 0 \right\} \to \{\sigma_{\rho,g} W_t, t \geq 0\}, \quad N \to \infty,$$

where

$$\sigma_{\rho,g}^2 = \sum_{k=p}^{\infty} g_k^2 k! \sum_{n \in \mathbb{Z}} \rho(n)^k.$$

As a corollary, we get asymptotic normality of the estimators. The statement depends on r, the order of filter a.

Theorem 5.3. *Let either $H \in (0, 3/4)$ or $H \in [3/4, 1)$ and $r \geq 2$. Then for any $m \geq 1$ the estimator $V_N^{a^m}$ is an asymptotically normal estimator of $\rho_H^{a^m}(0)$, and $\widehat{H}_N^{a,M}$ is an asymptotically normal estimator of H.*

Proof. We prove only the statement for $V_N^{a^m}$, the one for $\widehat{H}_N^{a,M}$ follows by writing explicitly the coefficient of linear regression and analyzing asymptotic expansions.
  Write

$$\sqrt{N - mq}\left(V_N^{a^m} - \rho_H^{a^m}(0)\right) = \frac{1}{\sqrt{N - mq}} \sum_{k=1}^{N-mq} \left((B_k^{a^m})^2 - \rho_H^{a^m}(0)\right)$$

$$= \frac{\rho_H^{a^m}(0)}{\sqrt{N - mq}} \sum_{k=1}^{N-mq} (\xi_k^2 - 1),$$

where $\xi_k = B_k^{a^m} / \sqrt{\rho_H^{a^m}(0)}$ is standard Gaussian. Obviously, $\rho(n) := \mathsf{E}\left[\xi_k \xi_{k+n}\right] = \rho^{a^m}(n)/\rho_H^{a^m}(0)$. Thus, we are in a position to apply the Breuer–Major theorem with $g(x) = x^2 - 1$, which is obviously of Hemrite rank 2. So we get the statement provided that $\sum_{n=1}^{\infty} \rho(n)^2 < \infty$. It was argued above that $\rho^{a^m}(n) \sim K_{H,a} m^{2H} n^{2(H-r)}, n \to +\infty$. Therefore, $\sum_{n=1}^{\infty} \rho(n)^2 < \infty$ iff $4(H - r) < -1$, equivalently, $r > H + 1/4$, which is exactly our assumption. $\qquad\square$

Remark 5.2. The last theorem can be used to construct approximate confidence intervals for H. It is possible to compute the asymptotic variance explicitly, but the expression for it is quite cumbersome, so it is not given here. A somewhat better approach is to numerically calculate it based on simulated data; the next section explains how to simulate fBm. Another observation is that the statement above depends on the value of H, which is a priori unknown and should be estimated. So, if one needs to construct a confidence interval for H, I suggest using a filter of order 2 unless it is *a priori* known that $H < 3/4$.

6. Simulation of Fractional Brownian Motion

Among many methods to simulate fBm, the most efficient one is probably the Wood–Chan, or circulant method. The main idea is that a Gaussian vector ξ with mean μ and covariance matrix C can be represented as $\xi = \mu + S\zeta$, where ζ is a standard Gaussian vector, and the matrix S is such that $SS^\top = C$. So in order to simulate a Gaussian vector, one needs to find a "square root" of covariance matrix.

Suppose that we need to simulate the values of fBm on some interval $[0, T]$. For practical purposes it is enough to simulate the values at a sufficiently fine grid, i.e. at the points $t_k^N = kT/N$, $k = 0, 1, \ldots, N$ for some large N. Since an fBm is self-similar and has stationary increments, it is enough to simulate the values $B_1^H, B_2^H, \ldots, B_N^H$ and multiply them by $(T/N)^H$. In turn, in order to simulate the latter values, it is suffices to simulate the increments $\xi_1 = B_1^H, \xi_2 = B_2^H - B_1^H, \ldots, \xi_N = B_N^H - B_{N-1}^H$. The random variables $\xi_1, \xi_2, \ldots, \xi_N$ form a stationary sequence of standard Gaussian variables with covariance

$$\rho_H(n) = \mathsf{E}\left[\xi_1 \xi_{n+1}\right] = \frac{1}{2}\left((n+1)^{2H} + (n-1)^{2H} - 2n^{2H}\right), \ n \geq 1;$$

this is so-called fractional Gaussian noise (fGn). In other words, $\xi = (\xi_1, \ldots, \xi_N)^\top$ is a centered Gaussian vector with covariance matrix

$$\mathrm{Cov}(\xi) = \begin{pmatrix} 1 & \rho_H(1) & \rho_H(2) & \cdots & \rho_H(N-2) & \rho_H(N-1) \\ \rho_H(1) & 1 & \rho_H(1) & \cdots & \rho_H(N-3) & \rho_H(N-2) \\ \rho_H(2) & \rho_H(1) & 1 & \cdots & \rho_H(N-4) & \rho_H(N-3) \\ \vdots & \vdots & \vdots & \ddots & \vdots & \vdots \\ \rho_H(N-2) & \rho_H(N-3) & \rho_H(N-4) & \cdots & 1 & \rho_H(1) \\ \rho_H(N-1) & \rho_H(N-2) & \rho_H(N-3) & \cdots & \rho_H(1) & 1 \end{pmatrix}.$$

Finding a square root of $\mathrm{Cov}(\xi)$ is not an easy task. It appears that one can much easier find a square root of some bigger matrix. Specifically, put $M = 2(N-1)$ and

$$c_0 = 1,$$
$$c_k = \begin{cases} \rho_H(k), & k = 1, 2, \ldots, N-1, \\ \rho_H(M-k), & k = N, N+1, \ldots, M-1. \end{cases} \tag{5}$$

Now define a circulant matrix

$$C = \mathrm{circ}(c_0, c_1, \ldots, c_{M-1}) = \begin{pmatrix} c_0 & c_1 & c_2 & \cdots & c_{M-2} & c_{M-1} \\ c_{M-1} & c_0 & c_1 & \cdots & c_{M-3} & c_{M-2} \\ c_{M-2} & c_{M-1} & c_0 & \cdots & c_{M-4} & c_{M-3} \\ \vdots & \vdots & \vdots & \ddots & \vdots & \vdots \\ c_2 & c_3 & c_4 & \cdots & c_0 & c_1 \\ c_1 & c_2 & c_3 & \cdots & c_{M-1} & c_0 \end{pmatrix}.$$

Now define a matrix $Q = (q_{jk})_{j,k=0}^{M-1}$, with

$$q_{jk} = \frac{1}{\sqrt{M}} \exp\left\{-2\pi i \frac{jk}{M}\right\}.$$

Observe that Q is unitary: $Q^*Q = QQ^* = I_M$, the identity matrix. The multiplication by matrix Q acts, up to the constant $1/\sqrt{M}$, as taking the discrete Fourier transform (DFT); the multiplication by Q^* is, up to the constant $\sqrt{M}$, taking the inverse DFT. The following statement easily follows from the properties of DFT and its inverse.

Theorem 6.1. *The circulant matrix C has a representation $C = Q\Lambda Q^*$, where $\Lambda = \mathrm{diag}(\lambda_0, \lambda_1, \ldots, \lambda_{M-1})$, $\lambda_k = \sum_{j=0}^{M-1} c_j \exp\left\{-2\pi i \frac{jk}{M}\right\}$. Consequently, $C = SS^*$ with $S = Q\Lambda^{1/2}Q^*$, $\Lambda^{1/2} = \mathrm{diag}(\lambda_0^{1/2}, \lambda_1^{1/2}, \ldots, \lambda_{M-1}^{1/2})$.*

The only problem with the last statement is that, generally speaking, the matrix S is complex. However, in the case of fBm the matrix C is positive definite, so all the eigenvalues λ_k are positive, as a result, the matrix S is real. Thus, in order to simulate the fGn, one needs to simulate a vector $(\zeta_1, \zeta_2, \ldots, \zeta_M)^\top$ of standard Gaussian variables, multiply it by S and take the first N coordinates of the resulting vector.

Let us turn to the practical realization of the algorithm. We start by noting that it is enough to compute the matrix S only once, then one can simulate as many realizations of fGn as needed. However, I do not recommend to proceed this way. It is usually better to compute the product $Q\Lambda^{1/2}Q^*\zeta$ step by step. First compute $\frac{1}{\sqrt{M}}Q^*\zeta$, taking the inverse DFT of ζ. Then multiply the result by $\Lambda^{1/2}$, i.e. multiply it elementwise by the vector $(\lambda_0^{1/2}, \lambda_1^{1/2}, \ldots, \lambda_{M-1}^{1/2})^\top$. The last step is the multiplication by $\sqrt{M}Q$, which is made by taking the DFT. As a result, we have one DFT computation, one elementwise multiplication, and one inverse DFT computation, which are usually faster than a single matrix multiplication.

Now it is a good moment to explain what is meant by "usually" in the last paragraph. It is well known that the DFT computation is most efficient when the size of data is a power of 2; it is made by the so-called fast Fourier transform (FFT) algorithm. So, if one needs to simulate e.g. $N = 1500$ values of fGn (so that $M = 2998$), it will be better (and faster) to simulate 2049 values (so that $M = 4096 = 2^{12}$).

Finally, taking in account everything said, we describe the algorithm.

1. Set $N = 2^q + 1$ and $M = 2^{q+1}$.
2. Calculate $\rho_H(1), \ldots, \rho_H(N-1)$ and set $c_0, c_1, \ldots, c_{M-1}$ according to (5).
3. Take FFT to get $\lambda_0, \ldots, \lambda_{M-1}$. Theoretically, one should get real numbers. However, since all computer calculations are imprecise, the resulting values will have tiny imaginary parts, so one needs to take the real part of result.
4. Generate independent standard Gaussian $\zeta_1, \ldots, \zeta_M$.

5. Take the real part of inverse FFT of $\zeta_1, \ldots, \zeta_M$ to obtain $\frac{1}{\sqrt{M}} Q^*(\zeta_1, \ldots, \zeta_M)^\top$.
6. Multiply the last elementwise by $\sqrt{\lambda_0}, \sqrt{\lambda_1}, \ldots, \sqrt{\lambda_{M-1}}$.
7. Take FFT of result to get

$$(\xi_1, \ldots, \xi_M)^\top = \sqrt{M} Q \Lambda^{1/2} \frac{1}{\sqrt{M}} Q^*(\zeta_1, \ldots, \zeta_M)^\top = S(\zeta_1, \ldots, \zeta_M)^\top.$$

8. Take the real part of $\xi_1, \ldots, \xi_N$ to get the fractional Gaussian noise.
9. Multiply by $(T/N)^H$ to obtain the increments of fBm.
10. Take cumulative sums to get the values of fBm.

For reader's convenience I give a Matlab code of (steps 1–8 of) this algorithm. It is split into two parts: the computation of $\Lambda^{1/2}$, which can be done only once, and the simulation.

```
function res = Lambda(H,N)
M = 2*N - 2;
C = zeros(1,M);
G = 2*H;
fbc = @(n)((n+1).^G + abs(n-1).^G - 2*n.^G)/2;
C(1:N) = fbc(0:(N-1));
C(N+1:M) = fliplr(C(2:(N-1)));
res = real(fft(C)).^0.5;


function res = FGN(lambda,NT)
if (~exist('NT','var'))
        NT = 1;
end
M = size(lambda,2);
a = bsxfun(@times,ifft(randn(NT,M),[],2),lambda);
res = real(fft(a,[],2));
res = res(:,1:(M/2));
```

To simulate n realizations of fGn, use the following code. Note that for large values of N and n, due to possible memory issues, it may be better to simulate the realizations one by one, using FGN(lambda,1) or simply FGN(lambda).

```
H = 0.7; q = 10; % or whatever you like
N = 2^q + 1;
lambda = Lambda(H,N);
n = 20; % or whatever you like
fGnsamples = FGN(lambda,20);
```

References

1. I. Nourdin, *Selected aspects of fractional Brownian motion*, Bocconi & Springer Series, Vol. 4 (Springer, Milan; Bocconi University Press, Milan, 2012).

2. D. Nualart, *The Malliavin calculus and related topics*, Probability and its Applications (New York), second edn. (Springer-Verlag, Berlin, 2006).
3. Y. S. Mishura, *Stochastic calculus for fractional Brownian motion and related processes*, Lecture Notes in Mathematics, Vol. 1929 (Springer-Verlag, Berlin, 2008).
4. F. Biagini, Y. Hu, B. Øksendal and T. Zhang, *Stochastic calculus for fractional Brownian motion and applications*, Probability and its Applications (New York) (Springer-Verlag London, Ltd., London, 2008).
5. J.-F. Coeurjolly, Simulation and identification of the fractional Brownian motion: a bibliographical and comparative study, *Journal of Statistical Software* **5**, 1 (2000).

7th Jagna International Workshop (2014)
International Journal of Modern Physics: Conference Series
Vol. 36 (2015) 1560003 (6 pages)
© The Author
DOI: 10.1142/S2010194515600034

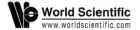

Local times for grey Brownian motion

J. L. da Silva

Centre of Exact Sciences and Engineering, University of Madeira,
Funchal, Madeira 9020-105, Portugal
luis@uma.pt
www.uma.pt

Published 2 January 2015

In this paper we study the grey Brownian motion, namely its representation and local time. First it is shown that grey Brownian motion may be represented in terms of a standard Brownian motion and then using a criterium of S. Berman, Trans. Amer. Math. Soc., **137**, 277–299 (1969), we show that grey Brownian motion admits a λ-square integrable local time almost surely (λ denotes the Lebesgue measure). As a consequence we obtain the occupation formula and state possible generalizations of these results.

Keywords: Brownian motion; grey Brownian motion; local time.

1. Introduction

Grey Brownian motion (gBm) was introduced by W. Schneider[1,2] as a model for slow anomalous diffusions, i.e., the marginal density function of the gBm is the fundamental solution of the time-fractional diffusion equation, see also Ref. 3. This is a class $\{B_\beta(t),\ t \geq 0,\ 0 < \beta \leq 1\}$ of processes which are self-similar with stationary increments. More recently, this class was extended to the, so called "generalized" grey Brownian motion (ggBm) to include slow and fast anomalous diffusions which contain either Gaussian or non-Gaussian processes e.g., fBm, gBm and others. The time evolution of the marginal density function of this class is described by partial integro-differential equations of fractional type, see Refs. 4,5. In this paper we investigate the class of gBm, namely their representation in terms of standard Brownian motion (Bm) and show the existence of local time.

In Section 2 we recall the construction and certain properties of gBm, in particular the representation of gBm as a product of Bm and an independent positive random variable, see (6) below. Here we would like to emphasize the fact that the representation (6) for gBm allow us to study certain properties of gBm in terms of those from Bm, e.g., path properties and simulations. Finally, in Section 3 we use the criterium due to S. Berman[6] in order to show that gBm admits a λ-square integrable local time, almost surely, cf. Theorem 3.1 below. As a corollary we obtain the occupation formula.

2. Grey Brownian motion

In this section we recall the construction of gBm due to W. Schneider.[2] The grey noise space is the probability space $(S'(\mathbb{R}), \mathcal{B}(S'(\mathbb{R})), \mu_\beta)$, where $S'(\mathbb{R})$ is the space of tempered distributions defined on $\mathbb{R}$, $\mathcal{B}(S'(\mathbb{R}))$ is the σ-algebra generated by the cylinder sets and μ_β is the grey noise measure given by its characteristic functional

$$\int_{S'(\mathbb{R})} e^{i\langle w, \varphi \rangle} \, d\mu_\beta(w) = E_\beta\left(-\frac{1}{2}\|\varphi\|^2\right), \quad \varphi \in S(\mathbb{R}), \ 0 < \beta \le 1. \tag{1}$$

Here $\langle \cdot, \cdot \rangle$ is the canonical bilinear pairing between $S(\mathbb{R})$ and $S'(\mathbb{R})$, $\|\cdot\|$ the norm in $L^2(\mathbb{R})$ and E_β is the Mittag-Leffler function of order β defined by

$$E_\beta(x) = \sum_{n=0}^{\infty} \frac{x^n}{\Gamma(\beta n + 1)}, \quad x \in \mathbb{R}.$$

The range $0 < \beta \le 1$ is to ensure the complete monotonicity of $E_\beta(-x)$, see Ref. 7, i.e., $(-1)^n E_\beta^{(n)}(-x) \ge 0$ for all $x \ge 0$ and $n \in \mathbb{N}_0 := \{0, 1, 2, \ldots\}$. In other words, there exists a probability measure ν_β on $\mathbb{R}_+$ which is absolutely continuous with respect to the Lebesgue measure with density M_β such that

$$E_\beta(-x) = \int_0^\infty e^{-\tau x} \, d\nu_\beta(\tau) = \int_0^\infty e^{-\tau x} M_\beta(\tau) \, d\tau. \tag{2}$$

The density M_β, the so-called M-Wright probability density function, is related to the fundamental solution of the time-fractional diffusion equation, emerges as a natural generalization of the Gaussian distribution. It is also a special case of the Wright function, namely, $M_\beta(x) = W_{-\beta, 1-\beta}(-x)$, see eq. (3.5) in Ref. 8.

The absolute moments of M_β in $\mathbb{R}_+$ are given by (see eq. (4.7) in Ref. 8)

$$\int_0^\infty \tau^\delta M_\beta(\tau) \, d\tau = \frac{\Gamma(\delta + 1)}{\Gamma(\beta \delta + 1)}, \quad \delta > -1. \tag{3}$$

Remark 2.1. Let μ_τ, $\tau > 0$, denote the Gaussian measure on $\mathcal{B}(S'(\mathbb{R}))$ with intensity τ, i.e.,

$$\int_{S'(\mathbb{R})} e^{i\langle w, \varphi \rangle} \, d\mu_\tau(w) = e^{-\frac{\tau}{2}\|\varphi\|^2}, \quad \varphi \in S(\mathbb{R}).$$

Then (2) gives the decomposition

$$\mu_\beta = \int_0^\infty \mu_\tau \, M_\beta(\tau) \, d\tau,$$

which says that the grey noise measure μ_β is the mixture of the the Gaussian measures μ_τ, $\tau \ge 0$ with $\mu_0 = \delta_0$ the Dirac measure at zero.

It is easy to show that the random variable $X_\beta(\mathbb{1}_{[0,t)})(\cdot) = \langle \cdot, \mathbb{1}_{[0,1)} \rangle$, $t \geq 0$ is a well defined element in $L^2(S'(\mathbb{R}), \mathcal{B}(S'(\mathbb{R})), \mu_\beta) =: L^2(\mu_\beta)$ and

$$\|X_\beta(\mathbb{1}_{[0,t)})\|^2_{L^2(\mu_\beta)} = \frac{1}{\Gamma(\beta+1)}\|\mathbb{1}_{[0,t)}\|^2 = \frac{1}{\Gamma(\beta+1)}t.$$

The gBm B_β is then defined as the stochastic process

$$B_\beta = \{B_\beta(t) := X_\beta(\mathbb{1}_{[0,t)}), \quad t \geq 0\}.$$

The following properties can be easily derived from (1) and the fact that $\|\mathbb{1}_{[0,t)}\|^2 = t$.

(1) $B_\beta(0) = 0$ almost surely. In addition, for each $t \geq 0$, the moments of any order are given by

$$\begin{cases} \mathbb{E}(B_\beta^{2n+1}(t)) &= 0 \\ \mathbb{E}(B_\beta^{2n}(t)) &= \frac{(2n)!}{2^n \Gamma(\beta n+1)}t^n. \end{cases}$$

Here $\mathbb{E}$ denotes the expectation with respect to μ_β.

(2) For each $t, s \geq 0$, the characteristic function of the increments is

$$\mathbb{E}\left(e^{i\theta(B_\beta(t)-B_\beta(s))}\right) = E_\beta\left(-\frac{\theta^2}{2}|t-s|\right), \quad \theta \in \mathbb{R}. \tag{4}$$

(3) The covariance function has the form

$$\mathbb{E}(B_\beta(t)B_\beta(s)) = \frac{1}{2\Gamma(\beta+1)}(t \wedge s), \quad t, s \geq 0. \tag{5}$$

All these properties may be summarized as follows. For any $0 < \beta \leq 1$, the gBm $B_\beta(t)$, $t \geq 0$, is $\frac{1}{2}$-self-similar with stationary increments. It is clear that for $\beta = 1$ the gBm coincides with Bm.

It was shown in Ref. 4 that the gBm B_β admits the following representation

$$\{B_\beta(t), \ t \geq 0\} \overset{d}{=} \{\sqrt{Y_\beta}B(t), \ t \geq 0\}, \tag{6}$$

where $\overset{d}{=}$ denotes the equality of the finite dimensional distribution and B is Bm. Y_β is an independent non-negative random variable with probability density function $M_\beta(\tau)$, $\tau \geq 0$.

3. Local times for grey Brownian motion

In this section we prove the existence of local times for gBm using the criterium due to Berman,[6] Lemma 3.1. For the readers convenience we recall the notion of occupation measure as well as occupation density.

Let $f : [0, T] \longrightarrow \mathbb{R}$ be a (nonrandom) measurable function and define, for any set $F \in \mathcal{B}(\mathbb{R})$, the occupation measure μ_f on $[0, T]$ of f up to "time" T by

$$\mu_f(F) := \int_I \mathbb{1}_F(f(s)) \, ds = \lambda(\{t \in [0, T] : f(t) \in F\}),$$

where λ is the Lebesgue measure on $[0, T]$. Hence, $\mu_f(F)$ describes the amount of time spent by f in F during the time period $[0, T]$. In particular, if $X = (X_t)_{t \in [0,T]}$ is a stochastic process, then the occupation measure of the sample path

$$[0, T] \ni t \mapsto X_t(w) \in \mathbb{R}$$

is defined in the same way but now the measure $\mu_{X.(w)}$ is a random measure, it depends on the sample point w of the probability space. We say that f has an occupation density over $[0, T]$ if μ_f is absolutely continuous with respect to the Lebesgue measure λ and denote this density by $L^f(\cdot, [0, T])$. In explicit form, for any $x \in \mathbb{R}$,

$$L^f(x, [0, T]) = \frac{d\mu_f}{d\lambda}(x).$$

Thus, we have

$$\mu_f(F) = \int_0^T \mathbb{1}_F(f(s)) \, ds = \int_F L^f(x, [0, T]) \, dx.$$

A continuous stochastic process X has an occupation density on $[0, T]$ if, for almost all $w \in \Omega$, $X.(w)$ has an occupation density $L^X(\cdot, [0, T])$, also called local time of X, see Berman.[6]

The criteria for the existence of local times for stochastic processes are due to Berman,[6] Section 3. More precisely, a stochastic process X admits a local time if and only if

$$\int_\mathbb{R} \left| \int_0^1 \int_0^1 \mathbb{E}\left(e^{i\theta(X(t)-X(s))}\right) ds \, dt \right| d\theta < \infty. \tag{7}$$

In the following we show that (7) is fulfilled if the stochastic process X is the gBm B_β. In fact, from (4) the characteristic function of the increments of gBm B_β is given by

$$\mathbb{E}\left(e^{i\theta(B_\beta(t)-B_\beta(s))}\right) = E_\beta\left(-\frac{\theta^2}{2}|t-s|\right).$$

Using Fubini, and the change of variables $r = (2)^{-1/2}\theta|t-s|^{1/2}$, we have to compute at first

$$\int_\mathbb{R} E_\beta\left(-\frac{\theta^2}{2}|t-s|\right) d\theta = \sqrt{\frac{2}{|t-s|}} \int_\mathbb{R} E_\beta(-r^2) \, dr.$$

The integral in the rhs may be computed using the representation of the Mittag-Leffler function (2), Fubini theorem again and the Gaussian integral, namely

$$\int_\mathbb{R} E_\beta(-r^2) \, dr = \int_0^\infty M_\beta(\tau) \int_\mathbb{R} e^{-r^2\tau} \, dr \, d\tau$$

$$= \sqrt{\pi} \int_0^\infty \tau^{-1/2} M_\beta(\tau) \, d\tau$$

$$= \sqrt{\pi} \frac{\Gamma(-\frac{1}{2}+1)}{\Gamma(-\beta\frac{1}{2}+1)}.$$

In the last equality we used the absolute moments of the M-Wright function M_β given in (3).

Finally, the t, s-integration is performed as follows.

$$\int_0^1 \int_0^1 \frac{1}{|t-s|^{1/2}} \, ds \, dt = 2 \int_0^1 \int_0^t \frac{1}{|t-s|^{1/2}} \, ds \, dt = 4 \int_0^1 t^{1/2} \, dt = \frac{8}{3}.$$

Therefore, putting all together, we obtain

$$\int_{\mathbb{R}} \left| \int_0^1 \int_0^1 \mathbb{E}\left(e^{i\theta(X(t)-X(s))}\right) \, ds \, dt \right| \, d\theta = \frac{8\sqrt{2\pi}}{3} \frac{\Gamma(-\frac{1}{2}+1)}{\Gamma(-\beta\frac{1}{2}+1)} < \infty.$$

Thus, we have shown the main result of this subsection which we state in the following theorem.

Theorem 3.1. *The gBm process B_β admits a λ-square integrable local time $L^{B_\beta}(\cdot, [0, T])$ almost surely.*

Corollary 3.1. *As a consequence of the existence of the local time $L^{B_\beta}(\cdot, [0, T])$, we obtain the occupation formula*

$$\int_0^T f(B_\beta(t)) \, dt = \int_{\mathbb{R}} f(x) L^{B_\beta}(x, [0, T]) \, dx, \quad a.s. \tag{8}$$

Remark 3.1. The above results may be generalized/realized in various directions.

(1) Theorem (3.1) may be generalized for the so-called "generalized" grey Brownian motion $B_{\beta,\alpha}$ introduced by A. Mura and F. Mainardi[5] such that for $\alpha = 1$ we recover the gBm, i.e., $B_{\beta,1} = B_\beta$. Moreover, the local times $L^{B_{\beta,\alpha}}(\cdot, [0, T])$ of $B_{\beta,\alpha}$ may be weak approximated by the number of crossings of a regularization by convolution of $B_{\beta,\alpha}$. For the details see Ref. 9.

(2) On the other hand, we may develop the Appell system which is a biorthogonal system of polynomials associated to the grey noise measure μ_β in order to construct, describe and characterize test and generalized functions spaces. Then the local time of gBm may be understood as a generalized function in this framework. For the details see Ref. 10.

Acknowledgments

Financial support of FCT through the research project PEst-OE/MAT/UI0219/ 2011. I would like to express my gratitude to Prof. M. Victoria Carpio-Bernido and Christopher C. Bernido as well as their team for the hospitality during my stay in Jagna for the 7th Jagna International Workshop.

References

1. W. R. Schneider, Grey noise, in *Stochastic processes, physics and geometry*, ed. S. Albeverio et al. (World Sci. Publ., Teaneck, NJ, 1990) pp. 676–681.
2. W. R. Schneider, Grey noise, in *Ideas and methods in mathematical analysis, stochastics, and applications (Oslo, 1988)*, eds. S. Albeverio, J. E. Fenstad, H. Holden and T. Lindstrøm (Cambridge Univ. Press, Cambridge, 1992) pp. 261–282.
3. W. R. Schneider, Fractional diffusion, in *Dynamics and stochastic processes (Lisbon, 1988)*, eds. R. Lima, L. Streit and R. V. Mendes, Lecture Notes in Phys., Vol. 355 (Springer, New York, 1990) pp. 276–286.
4. A. Mura and G. Pagnini, Characterizations and simulations of a class of stochastic processes to model anomalous diffusion, *J. Phys. A* **41**, 285003, 22 (2008).
5. A. Mura and F. Mainardi, A class of self-similar stochastic processes with stationary increments to model anomalous diffusion in physics, *Integral Transforms Spec. Funct.* **20**, 185 (2009).
6. S. M. Berman, Local times and sample function properties of stationary Gaussian processes, *Trans. Amer. Math. Soc.* **137**, 277 (1969).
7. H. Pollard, The completely monotonic character of the Mittag-Leffler function $E_a(-x)$, *Bull. Amer. Math. Soc.* **54**, 1115 (1948).
8. F. Mainardi, A. Mura and G. Pagnini, The M-Wright function in time-fractional diffusion processes: A tutorial survey, *Int. J. Differ. Equ.* **2010**, Art. ID 104505, 29 (2010).
9. J. L. Da Silva and M. Erraoui, Grey Brownian motion local time: Existence and weak-approximation, *To appear in Stochastics* (2014).
10. M. Grothaus, F. Jahnert, F. Riemann and J. L. Silva, Mittag-Leffler analysis I. Construction, description and characterization, In preparation, (2014).

7th Jagna International Workshop (2014)
International Journal of Modern Physics: Conference Series
Vol. 36 (2015) 1560004 (16 pages)
© The Authors
DOI: 10.1142/S2010194515600046

World Scientific
www.worldscientific.com

Adapted integral representations of random variables

Georgiy Shevchenko

Department of Mechanics and Mathematics,
Taras Shevchenko National University of Kyiv
Volodymirska 60, 01601 Kyiv, Ukraine
zhora@univ.kiev.ua

Lauri Viitasaari

Department of Mathematics and System Analysis,
Aalto University School of Science, Helsinki
P. O. Box 11100, FIN-00076 Aalto, Finland
lauri.viitasaari@aalto.fi

Published 2 January 2015

We study integral representations of random variables with respect to general Hölder continuous processes and with respect to two particular cases; fractional Brownian motion and mixed fractional Brownian motion. We prove that an arbitrary random variable can be represented as an improper integral, and that the stochastic integral can have any distribution. If in addition the random variable is a final value of an adapted Hölder continuous process, then it can be represented as a proper integral. It is also shown that in the particular case of mixed fractional Brownian motion, any adapted random variable can be represented as a proper integral.

Keywords: Hölder processes; fractional Brownian motion; mixed fractional Brownian motion; pathwise integral; generalized Lebesgue–Stieltjes integral; integral representation.

1. Introduction

Let $(\Omega, \mathcal{F}, \mathbb{F} = \{\mathcal{F}_t, t \in [0,1]\}, P)$ be a stochastic basis, and $\{X(t), t \in [0,1]\}$ be an $\mathbb{F}$-adapted process.

We consider representations of the form

$$\xi = \int_0^1 \psi(s)\mathrm{d}X(s), \tag{1.1}$$

where ϕ is an $\mathbb{F}$-adapted process and ξ some given $\mathcal{F}_1$-measurable random variable.

While such representation also has theoretical interest the question is particularly motivated by mathematical finance. Indeed, ξ can be viewed as the claim to be hedged and the integral representation corresponds to the value of the hedging portfolio. However, there is a constant representing the value of the claim missing in equation (1.1). Consequently, claims ξ with representation (1.1) can be hedged with zero cost. In particular, the results presented in this paper indicates that models where the stock process $X(t)$ is Hölder continuous of some order $\alpha > \frac{1}{2}$ are rarely good models since there will be arbitrage present with relatively simple trading strategies ψ.

The representations similar to (1.1) were considered by many authors, we cite here only the most relevant results. The first results of this kind were established for $X = W$, the standard Wiener process. In this case, the classical Itô representation theorem provides the representation (1.1) for square integrable centered random variables ξ with the integrand satisfying $\int_0^1 \mathbb{E}\psi(t)^2 dt < \infty$. Such representation was shown to take place for any random variable ξ in Ref. 1, but with integrand satisfying $\int_0^1 \psi(t)^2 dt < \infty$ a.s. The case where $X = B^H$, a fractional Brownian motion with $H \in (1/2, 1)$, was considered first in Ref. 2. Under assumption that there exists a Hölder continuous adapted process $\{z(t), t \in [0,1]\}$ such that $z(1) = \xi$, it was shown that ξ can be represented in the form (1.1). In Ref. 3 this result was extended to a larger class of Gaussian processes, and in Ref. 4, under a similar assumption, the existence of representation (1.1) with integrand $\psi \in C[0,1)$ was established.

In this article we generalize the results of both Ref. 3 and Ref. 4 by showing the existence of the representation (1.1) with $\psi \in C[0,1)$ for a generic Hölder continuous process X satisfying some small ball estimates. We also show that in the case of mixed fractional Brownian motion, i.e. where $X = W + B^H$, the representation (1.1) takes place for any random variable ξ. The structure of the article is as follows. Section 2 contains basic information on the generalized Lebesgue–Stieltjes integral. Section 3 is devoted to the auxiliary construction of processes which play an important role in proving the main representation results. Section 4 contains the main results concerning the representation of random variables.

2. Generalized Lebesgue–Stieltjes Integral

This section gives a basic information on the generalized Lebesgue–Stieltjes integral, more details can be found in Ref. 5. For functions $f, g \colon [a, b] \to \mathbb{R}$ and $\beta \in (0, 1)$, define the fractional derivatives

$$\left(D_{a+}^{\beta} f\right)(x) = \frac{1}{\Gamma(1-\beta)} \left(\frac{f(x)}{(x-a)^{\beta}} + \beta \int_a^x \frac{f(x) - f(u)}{(x-u)^{\beta+1}} du \right),$$

$$\left(D_{b-}^{1-\beta} g\right)(x) = \frac{e^{-i\pi\beta}}{\Gamma(\beta)} \left(\frac{g(x)}{(b-x)^{1-\beta}} + (1-\beta) \int_x^b \frac{g(x) - g(u)}{(u-x)^{2-\beta}} du \right).$$

Assuming that $D_{a+}^{\beta} f \in L_1[a,b]$, $D_{b-}^{1-\beta} g_{b-} \in L_\infty[a,b]$, where $g_{b-}(x) = g(x) - g(b)$, the generalized Lebesgue-Stieltjes integral $\int_a^b f(x) dg(x)$ is defined as

$$\int_a^b f(x)\mathrm{d}g(x) = e^{i\pi\beta}\int_a^b \left(D_{a+}^\beta f\right)(x)\left(D_{b-}^{1-\beta}g_{b-}\right)(x)\mathrm{d}x.$$

¿From the definition, we have an immediate estimate

$$\left|\int_a^b f(x)\mathrm{d}g(x)\right| \le C\|f\|_{\beta;[a,b]}\Lambda_\beta(g), \tag{2.1}$$

where

$$\|f\|_{\beta;[a,b]} = \int_a^b \left(\frac{f(t)}{(t-a)^\beta} + \int_a^t \frac{|f(t)-f(s)|}{(t-s)^{\beta+1}}\mathrm{d}s\right)\mathrm{d}t,$$

$$\Lambda_\beta(g) = \sup_{a\le u<v\le b} \left(\frac{|g(v)-g(u)|}{(v-u)^{1-\beta}} + \int_u^v \frac{|g(u)-g(z)|}{(z-u)^{2-\beta}}\mathrm{d}z\right).$$

Here and in the rest of the article we will use the symbol C to denote a positive constant, whose value is of no importance and may change from one line to another.

It is easy to see that if g is α-Hölder continuous on $[a,b]$ and $\beta \in (1-\alpha,1)$, then $\Lambda_\beta(g) < \infty$. Therefore, it is possible to define $\int_a^b f(x)\mathrm{d}g(x)$ in the generalized Lebesgue–Stieltjes sense once the integrand f satisfies $\|f\|_{\beta;[a,b]} < \infty$. In what follows we will consider the functions satisfying this condition to be our admissible integrands.

3. Adapted Processes Which Integrate to Infinity

At the heart of each representation lies an auxiliary construction of an adapted integrand ψ such that for each $t < 1$ the integral $v_t(\psi) := \int_0^t \psi(s)\mathrm{d}X(s)$ is finite, but the integral $\int_0^1 \psi(s)\mathrm{d}X(s)$ is infinite. The latter property can have different precise meanings: either $v_t(\psi) \to +\infty, t \to 1-$ or $\liminf_{t\to 1-} v_t(\psi) = -\infty$, $\limsup_{t\to 1-} v_t(\psi) = +\infty$.

3.1. *Construction in a generic case*

To obtain such auxiliary construction for a general process there are essentially two key features which we study here; the process is assumed to be Hölder continuous for some order $\alpha > 1/2$ and there should be some kind of estimate for small ball probability for the increment of the process. We also wish to emphasize that these properties are needed only close to the end point $t = 1$ (or more generally, $t = T$). Consequently, the replication procedure can be done in arbitrary small amount of time. This can be useful for example in financial applications since one can simply wait and observe the process and study whether it might indeed have the needed properties, and then start the replication procedure just before the ending point. For more detailed discussion in the Gaussian case we refer to Ref. 3.

Assumption 1. There exist a constants $\alpha > \frac{1}{2}$ such that for every $s,t \in [0,1]$ it holds

$$|X(t) - X(s)| \le C\,|t-s|^\alpha .$$

Assumption 2. There exists a constant $\delta > 0$ such that for every $s, t \in [1 - \delta, 1]$ with $t = s + \Delta$ it holds

$$\mathbb{P}(\sup_{s \leq u \leq t} |X(u) - X(s)| \leq \epsilon) \leq \exp\left(-C\Delta\epsilon^{-\frac{1}{\alpha}}\right) \tag{3.1}$$

provided that $\epsilon \leq \Delta^\alpha$.

Note that the given upper bound for small ball probability is the usual one for many Gaussian processes and hence we wish to use this form. For example, many stationary Gaussian processes or Gaussian processes with stationary increments satisfy the given assumption. In particular, fractional Brownian motion satisfies the given assumption. For more detailed discussion on the assumption, see.[3] We also remark that by examining our proofs below it is clear that one could relax the assumption by giving less sharp upper bound in terms of Δ and ϵ (see Remark 3.1).

Lemma 3.1. *Assume that the process X satisfies Assumptions 1 and 2. Then there exists a $\mathbb{F}$-adapted continuous process ϕ on $[0,1)$ such that $\phi(0) = 0$, the integral*

$$\int_0^t \phi(s)\mathrm{d}X(s)$$

exists for every $t < 1$ and

$$\lim_{t \to 1-} \int_0^t \phi(s)\mathrm{d}X(s) = +\infty \tag{3.2}$$

almost surely.

It turns out that the construction presented in the particular case of fBm in the authors' previous work[4] works for general Hölder continuous processes under our small ball Assumption 2. Hence we simply present the key points of the proof.

Proof. Fix numbers $\gamma \in \left(1, \frac{1}{\alpha}\right)$, $\eta \in \left(0, \frac{1}{\gamma\alpha} - 1\right)$ and $\mu > \frac{1}{\alpha(1+\eta)}$. Set $t_0 = 0$ and $t_n = \sum_{k=1}^n (\Delta_k + \tilde{\Delta}_k)$, where $\Delta_k = Kk^{-\gamma}$, $\tilde{\Delta}_k = Kk^{-\mu}$, $K = \left(\sum_{k=1}^\infty (k^{-\gamma} + k^{-\mu})\right)^{-1}$. Also set $t_n' = t_{n-1} + \Delta_n$, $n \geq 1$. Clearly, $t_{n-1} < t_n' < t_n$, $n \geq 1$, and $t_n \to 1$, $n \to \infty$. Note also that if X_t would be α-Hölder only close to the end point, i.e. on $[1 - \delta, 1]$ for some small δ, then we simply set $t_1 = 1 - \delta$ such that X is Hölder on $[t_1, 1]$ and start after t_1 by scaling time points properly. This also implies that the construction can be done in arbitrary small amount of time.

Next define the sequence of functions $g_n = \sqrt{x^2 + n^{-2}} - n^{-1}$, $n \geq 1$. Then $g_n(x) \uparrow |x|$, $n \to \infty$. Let also $f_n = (1 + \eta)g_n(x)^\eta \frac{x}{\sqrt{x^2+n^{-2}}}$ so that $g_n(x)^{1+\eta} = \int_0^x f_n(z)\mathrm{d}z$. For any $n \geq 1$ set

$$\tau_n = \min\left\{t \geq t_{n-1} : |X(t) - X(t_{n-1})| \geq n^{-1/(1+\eta)}\right\} \wedge t_n'.$$

Next define

$$\phi(s) = f_n(X(s) - X(t_{n-1}))\mathbf{1}_{[t_{n-1}, \tau_n)}(s)$$

for $s \in [t_{n-1}, \tau_n]$ and

$$\phi(s) = \phi(\tau_n) \frac{\tau_n + \widetilde{\Delta}_n - s}{\widetilde{\Delta}_n} \mathbf{1}_{(\tau_n, \tau_n + \widetilde{\Delta}_n]}(s)$$

for $s \in (\tau_n, t_n]$. Now by Hölder continuity of X the existence of the integral is clear, and we can repeat the arguments in Ref. 4 to obtain that

$$\int_0^{t_n} \phi(s) dX(s) \geq 2^{-\eta} \sum_{k=1}^n |X(\tau_k) - X(t_{k-1})|^{1+\eta}$$
$$- \sum_{k=1}^n k^{-1-\eta}$$
$$+ \sum_{k=1}^n \int_{\tau_k}^{\tau_k + \widetilde{\Delta}_k} \phi(s) dX(s).$$

Moreover, it is clear that the second sum converges and arguments in Ref. 4 imply that also the third sum converges by Hölder continuity of X. To conclude, the Assumption 2 implies that the first sum diverges since now only a finite number of events

$$A_n = \{ \sup_{t_{n-1} \leq t \leq t'_n} |X(t) - X(t_{n-1})| < n^{-1/(1+\eta)} \}$$

happens by Borel–Cantelli Lemma and Assumption 2. Hence the result follows. □

Remark 3.1. By Assumption 2 we obtain that

$$\mathbb{P}(A_n) \leq \exp\left(-C n^{\frac{1}{\alpha(1+\beta)} - \gamma}\right)$$

for some constant C. Hence it is clear that our assumption on small ball probabilities could be relaxed a lot. In particular, we only need that

$$\sum_{n=1}^{\infty} \mathbb{P}(A_n) < \infty$$

to apply Borel–Cantelli lemma.

3.2. *Construction in pure and mixed fractional Brownian cases*

In this section we consider two important particular cases: $X = B^H$, a fractional Brownian motion with $H > 1/2$ and $X = B^H + W$, a mixed fractional Brownian motion. We start with the pure fractional Brownian case.

Lemma 3.2. *Let* $f(t) = (1-t)^{-H}$, $v(t) = \int_0^t f(s) dB^H(s)$. *Then* $\liminf_{t \to 1-} v(t) = -\infty$, $\limsup_{t \to 1-} v(t) = +\infty$ *almost surely.*

Proof. Define $x_n = v(1-2^{-n}) - v(1-2^{-n+1})$, $n \geq 1$. Then the sequence $\{x_n, n \geq 1\}$ is stationary Gaussian. Indeed, for any $m \geq n \geq 1$,

$$
\begin{aligned}
\mathbb{E}x_n x_m &= \alpha_H \int_{1-2^{-n+1}}^{1-2^{-n}} \int_{1-2^{-m+1}}^{1-2^{-m}} |u-v|^{2H-2}(1-u)^{-H}(1-v)^{-H} \mathrm{d}u \, \mathrm{d}v \\
&= \alpha_H \int_{2^{-n}}^{2^{-n+1}} \int_{2^{-m}}^{2^{-m+1}} |y-x|^{2H-2} x^{-H} y^{-H} \mathrm{d}x \, \mathrm{d}y \\
&= \alpha_H \int_{1}^{2} \int_{2^{n-m}}^{2^{n-m+1}} |2^{-n}z - 2^{-n}w|^{2H-2} 2^{nH} w^{-H} 2^{nH} z^{-H} 2^{-n} \mathrm{d}w \, 2^{-n} \mathrm{d}z \\
&= \alpha_H \int_{1}^{2} \int_{2^{n-m}}^{2^{n-m+1}} |z-w|^{2H-2} w^{-H} z^{-H} \mathrm{d}w \, \mathrm{d}z = r(n-m),
\end{aligned}
$$

where $\alpha_H = H(2H-1)$. Moreover, it is clear that $r(k) = O(2^{k(1-H)})$, $k \to \infty$. Therefore, defining $S_n = x_1 + x_2 + \cdots + x_n$, $n \to \infty$, we have $\limsup_{n\to\infty} S_n = +\infty$, $\liminf_{n\to\infty} S_n = -\infty$ a.s. by the law of iterated logarithm for weakly dependent stationary sequences. Observing that $v(1-2^{-n}) = S_n$, we get the statement. □

Further we move to the case of a mixed fractional Brownian motion. This means that $X = B^H + W$, where B^H is a fractional Brownian motion with $H \in (1/2, 1)$, and W is a standard Wiener process. Usually it is assumed that B^H and W are independent, but we do not impose any assumptions of such kind. Note that we understand the integral w.r.t. the standard Wiener process W in the classical Itô sense and the integral w.r.t. B^H in the generalized Lebesgue–Stieltjes sense.

The following lemma provides an "auxiliary" construction in this case and even if it will not be used in the following, we give it for two reasons: to make our presentation complete and to disclose the main idea behind the proof of our main result in the mixed case.

Lemma 3.3. *Let* $f(t) = (1-t)^{-1/2}$, $v(t) = \int_0^t f(s)\mathrm{d}(W(s) + B^H(s))$. *Then* $\liminf_{t\to 1-} v(t) = -\infty$, $\limsup_{t\to 1-} v(t) = +\infty$ *almost surely.*

Proof. Define $u(t) = \int_0^t f(s)\mathrm{d}W(s)$. Then it is easy to see that u has the same distribution as the time-changed Wiener process, $\{u(t), t \in [0,1]\} \overset{d}{=} \{W(-\ln(1-t)), t \in [0,1]\}$. Hence we get by the law of iterated logarithm $\liminf_{t\to 1-} u(t) = -\infty$, $\limsup_{t\to 1+} u(t) = +\infty$. So it remains to prove that the integral $\int_0^t (1-s)^{-1/2} \mathrm{d}B^H(s)$ is bounded. But the integrand is non-random, so the integral coincides with the so-called Wiener integral, and its boundedness follows from the finiteness of

$$
\begin{aligned}
\mathbb{E}\left(\int_0^1 f(s)\mathrm{d}B^H(s) \right)^2 \\
= H(2H-1) \int_0^1 \int_0^1 (1-t)^{-1/2}(1-s)^{-1/2} |t-s|^{2H-2} \mathrm{d}u \, \mathrm{d}s \\
= 2H \, \mathrm{B}(2H-1, 1/2).
\end{aligned}
$$

□

4. Representation of Random Variables

In the case of fBm it was shown in Ref. 2 that the integral $\int_0^1 \phi(s)\mathrm{d}B^H(s)$ can have any distribution and later in Ref. 3 the same result was proved for wider class of Gaussian processes. Similarly, any random variable can be represented as an improper integral in these models. These results are a consequence of the auxiliary construction and hence we can obtain similar results by applying the auxiliary construction introduced in the previous section for any Hölder process which has some small ball estimates. More precisely, a direct consequence of Lemma 3.1 is that the integral can have any distribution and if in addition we have diverging auxiliary construction on any (suitable) subinterval, then any measurable random variable can be represented as an improper integral. These results are the topic of the next theorems.

Theorem 4.1. *Let the process $X(t)$ satisfy Assumptions 1, 2, and let there exist $v \in (1 - \delta, 1)$ such that the random variable $X(v)$ has continuous distribution. Then for any distribution function F there exists a $\mathbb{F}$-adapted process φ such that the integral*

$$\int_0^1 \varphi(s)\mathrm{d}X(s)$$

exists and has distribution F.

Proof. Since $X(v)$ has continuous distribution with cdf F_X, then $U = F_X(X(v))$ is uniformly distributed random variable and consequently, $F^{-1}(U)$ has distribution F. Hence it suffices to construct φ such that

$$\int_0^1 \varphi(s)\mathrm{d}X(s) = F^{-1}[F_X(X(v))].$$

Denote by $g(x) = F^{-1}[F_X(x)]$. Let ϕ be the process constructed in Lemma 3.1 and set $y_t = \int_v^t \phi(s)\mathrm{d}X(s)$. Then $y_t \to \infty$ as $t \to 1-$. Put $\tau = \inf\{t \geq v : y_t = |g(X(v))|\}$ and

$$\varphi(t) = \phi(t)\operatorname{sgn} g(X(v))\mathbf{1}_{[v,\tau]}.$$

Clearly $\int_0^1 \varphi(s)\mathrm{d}X(s)$ has distribution F and the existence of integral is obvious from which the result follows. $\qquad\square$

To replicate a distribution we needed an additional assumption that $X(v)$ has continuous distribution for some v. Similarly, in order to replicate an arbitrary random variable we need a different additional assumption. Namely, we assume that the filtration $\mathbb{F}$ is left-continuous at 1, i.e. $\sigma(\bigcup_{t<1} \mathcal{F}_t) = \mathcal{F}_1$.

Theorem 4.2. *Assume that $\mathbb{F}$ is left-continuous at 1 and let the process X satisfy Assumptions 1 and 2. Then for any $\mathcal{F}_1$-measurable random variable ξ there exists a process $\psi(s)$ such that*

$$\int_0^t \psi(s)\mathrm{d}X(s)$$

exists for every $t < 1$ and

$$\lim_{t \to 1} \int_0^t \psi(s)\mathrm{d}X(s) = \xi \tag{4.1}$$

almost surely.

Proof. Note first that by modifying the proof of Lemma 3.1 we see that Assumption 2 implies the existence of auxiliary construction on every subinterval $[u, v] \subset [1 - \delta, 1]$, i.e. for every such interval there exists a process $\phi_{u,v}$ such that $\lim_{t \to v} \int_u^v \phi_{u,v}(s)\mathrm{d}X(s) = \infty$. The rest follows by arguments in Ref. 2 and we only present the main steps. Define $z(t) = \tan \mathbb{E}[\arctan \xi | \mathcal{F}_t]$. Now by left-continuity of $\mathbb{F}$ and martingale convergence theorem we have $z(t) \to \xi$, $t \to 1-$. Let next t_n be arbitrary increasing sequence converging to 1, and let $\phi_{t_n,t_{n+1}}$ be a process constructed in Lemma 3.1 such that $v_t^n = \int_{t_n}^t \phi_{t_n,t_{n+1}}(s)\mathrm{d}X(s) \to \infty$ as $t \to t_{n+1}-$. Defining $\tau_n = \min\{t \geq t_n : v_t^n = |z(t_n) - z(t_{n-1})|\}$ and

$$\psi(s) = \sum_{n=1}^{\infty} \phi_{t_n,t_{n+1}}(s)\mathbf{1}_{[t_n,\tau_n]}(s)\mathrm{sign}(z(t_n) - z(t_{n-1}))$$

it is clear that $\int_0^{t_n} \psi(s)\mathrm{d}X(s) = z(t_{n-1})$ and on $t \in [t_n, t_{n+1}]$ the value $\int_0^t \psi(s)\mathrm{d}X(s)$ is between $z(t_{n-1})$ and $z(t_n)$. Hence it follows that we have (4.1). The existence of the integral can be shown as in the proof of Lemma 3.1. $\square$

Remark 4.1. We remark that it is also possible to construct a continuous process ψ on $[0, 1)$ such that $\lim_{t \to 1} \int_0^t \psi(s)\mathrm{d}X(s) = \xi$ by applying similar techniques as in Ref. 4 or in the proof of Theorem 4.3. More precisely, after stopping τ_n let $\psi(s)$ go to zero linearly on $t \in [\tau_n, \tau_n + \Delta_n]$ for small enough Δ_n, and then compensate the error arising from linear parts by setting $\tau_n = \min\{t \geq t_n : v_t^n = |z(t_n) - z(t_{n-1}) - \int_{\tau_{n-1}}^{\tau_{n-1}+\Delta_n} \psi(s)\mathrm{d}X(s)|\}$. The details are left to the reader.

A particularly interesting question for us is which random variables can be represented as a proper integral.

4.1. *A proper representation in a generic case*

It turns out that with general Hölder process satisfying our small ball assumption one can represent all random variables that can be viewed as an end value of some a-Hölder process with arbitrary $a > 0$. In the particular case of fBm this was proved first in Ref. 2. Similar result for more general Gaussian process was derived in Ref. 3. However, in this case it was proved that only values $a > 1 - \alpha$ can be covered where α is the Hölder index of the process X. The benefit of using continuous integrands is that then one can drop unnecessary extra assumptions. Moreover, then one can cover all values of $a > 0$ also in the case of general Gaussian process. More precisely, in the author's previous work[4] it was proved that in the case of fBm one can construct a continuous integrand Ψ on $[0, 1)$ such that

$$\xi = \int_0^1 \Psi(s)\mathrm{d}B^H(s).$$

By examining the proof however, we obtain that only required facts are Hölder continuity, small ball estimate and the auxiliary construction with continuous integrand. Hence the arguments presented in Ref. 4 imply same result for our general case. Note also that, as before, the replication can be done in arbitrary small amount of time and the assumed properties are needed only close to the ending point $t = 1$.

Theorem 4.3. *Let the process $X(t)$ satisfy Assumptions 1 and 2. Furthermore, assume there exists an $\mathbb{F}$-adapted process $\{z(t), t \geq 0\}$ having Hölder continuous paths of order $a > 0$ and such that $z(1) = \xi$. Then there exists an $\mathbb{F}$-adapted process $\{\psi(t), t \in [0, 1]\}$ such that $\psi \in C[0, 1)$ a.s. and*

$$\int_0^1 \psi(s)\mathrm{d}X(s) = \xi \tag{4.2}$$

almost surely.

The proof follows arguments presented in Ref. 4 but here we will give more instructive proof while some technical steps are omitted.

The idea of the proof is to define a sequence of time points $(t_n)_{n=0}^\infty$ converging to 1 and then track the Hölder process $z(t)$ along this sequence such that

$$\int_0^{t_n} \psi(s)\mathrm{d}X(s) = z(t_{n-1}). \tag{4.3}$$

More precisely, we apply our diverging auxiliary construction to "get into the right track", and afterwards we aim to stay on this right track. Now there are two options; given that we have (4.3) for some n we either manage to stay on the right track and consequently we have (4.3) also for $n + 1$ or if we do not, then we apply the auxiliary construction together with stopping again to get "back to the track". Note that while we could apply the auxiliary construction separately on every interval $[t_{n-1}, t_n]$, consequently the integral $\int_0^1 \psi(s)\mathrm{d}X(s)$ over the whole interval would not exist. Hence to obtain the result we simply have to show that we indeed manage to stay on the right path in most of the cases, and the auxiliary construction is needed only finite number of times. Finally, in order to construct a continuous integrand we simply pace to zero linearly after every time step before starting to act on the next time interval.

Proof of Theorem 4.3. Choose some $\beta \in (1 - \alpha, 1)$. Let Δ_k be sequence such that $\sum_{k=1}^\infty \Delta_k = 1$ and define time points $t_0 = 0$, $t_n = \sum_{k=1}^n \Delta_k$. Set also $t'_n = t_{n-1} + \frac{\Delta_n}{2}$. Note that now $t_{n-1} < t'_n < t_n$. Let also $\widetilde{\Delta}_k$ be a sequence to be determined later such that $\widetilde{\Delta}_k \leq \frac{\Delta_k}{2}$. Following the idea described above, our aim is to define continuous integrand such that we track the process $z(t)$ on intervals $[t_{n-1}, t'_n]$ and then we go linearly to zero such that the integrand hits zero before time t_{n+1}. Then on $[t_{n+1}, t'_{n+1}]$ we define continuous integrand ψ such that $\psi(t_{n+1}) = 0$ and we are tracking the process $z(t)$. Note also that on every step we have to compensate the error arising from linear parts. We will first explain naively the construction which is somewhat simple. The end of the proof is devoted to analysis on different parameters where we show that one can indeed choose them such that we obtain our result.

Step 1. Construction. We start by setting $\psi(t) = 0$ on the interval $[t_0, t_1]$. Moreover, we set $\tau_1 = t_1$.

Denote $y(t) = \int_0^t \psi(s) dX(s)$, $\xi_n = z(t_{n-1})$, $g_n(x) = \sqrt{x^2 + \epsilon_n^2} - \epsilon_n$ for some sequence ϵ_n and let now $n \geq 2$. To describe our construction mathematically, we want to define the process ψ on $[t_{n-1}, t_n]$ such that

(1) $\psi(t_{n-1}) = \psi(t_n) = 0$;
(2) $y(\tau_n) = \xi_n$ for some $\tau_n \in [t_n, t'_n]$;
(3) ψ is linear on $[\tau_n, \tau_n + \widetilde{\Delta}_n]$ and zero afterwards, i.e.

$$\psi(t) = \psi(\tau_n) \frac{\tau_n + \widetilde{\Delta}_n - t}{\widetilde{\Delta}_n} \mathbf{1}_{(\tau_n, \tau_n + \widetilde{\Delta}_n]}(t), \quad t \in [\tau_n, t_n]. \qquad (4.4)$$

Now the construction is different whether we are already "on the right path" (case A) or not (case B) in which case we apply the auxiliary construction of Lemma 3.1.

Case A) $y(\tau_{n-1}) = \xi_{n-1}$. For a sequence a_n to be determined later, define

$$\tau_n = \inf \left\{ t \geq t_{n-1} : a_n g_n(X(t) - X(t_{n-1})) = |\Lambda_n| \right\} \wedge t'_n,$$

where $\Lambda_n = \xi_n - y(t_{n-1}) = \xi_n - \xi_{n-1} - \int_{\tau_{n-1}}^{t_{n-1}} \psi(s) dX(s)$. Put

$$\psi(t) = a_n g'_n(X(t) - X(t_{n-1})) \operatorname{sign} \Lambda_n, \quad t \in [t_{n-1}, \tau_n]$$

and define it by (4.4) on $[\tau_n, t_n]$. Now since $X(t)$ is Hölder continuous of order $\alpha > \frac{1}{2}$, it obeys the classical change of variable rule. Hence we get

$$y(t) = y(t_{n-1}) + a_n g_n(X(t) - X(t_{n-1})) \operatorname{sign} \Lambda_n, \quad t \in [t_{n-1}, \tau_n];$$

in particular, $y(\tau_n) = \xi_n$ provided that $\tau_n < t'_n$.

Case B) $y(\tau_{n-1}) \neq \xi_{n-1}$. Since Assumption 2 implies that there exists diverging auxiliary construction also on every subinterval, there exists an adapted continuous process $\{\phi_n(t), t \in [t_{n-1}, t'_n]\}$ such that $v_n(t) := \int_{t_n}^t \phi_n(s) dX(s) \to \infty$, $t \to t'_n-$. Therefore we can define the stopping time $\tau_n = \inf\{t \in [t_{n-1}, t'_n) : v(t) = |\xi_n - y(\tau_{n-1})|\}$. Then we put $\psi(t) = \phi_n(t) \operatorname{sign}(\xi_n - y(\tau_{n-1}))$, $t \in [t_{n-1}, \tau_n]$, and use (4.4) on $[\tau_n, t_n]$. Clearly, $y(\tau_n) = \xi_n$.

Step 2. "Staying on the right path" and continuity of the integral. To obtain our result we wish to apply Assumption 2 to obtain that we have Case A) in most of the cases and that representation (4.2) holds. For the latter one, it is sufficient to prove that the integral $\int_0^t \psi(s) dX(s)$ is continuous at $t = 1$ which also implies the existence of the integral. Consequently, we end up to some restrictions on free parameters. Similarly, note that in order to prove that we have Case A) in most of the cases we have to prove that the event

$$A_n = \left\{ \sup_{t \in [t_{n-1}, t'_n)} a_n g_n (X(t) - X(t_{n-1})) \le |\Lambda_n| \right\}$$

happens only finite number of times. Now by following arguments in Ref. 4 we obtain $|\psi(\tau_{n-1})| \le a_n$ for every n and

$$\left| \int_{\tau_{n-1}}^{t_{n-1}} \psi(s) dX(s) \right| \le C_\epsilon(\omega) |\phi(\tau_{n-1})| \widetilde{\Delta}_{n-1}^{\alpha-\epsilon} \le C_\epsilon(\omega) a_n \widetilde{\Delta}_{n-1}^{\alpha-\epsilon}$$

by Hölder continuity of X. Moreover, observing that $g_{\epsilon_n}(x) \ge |x| - \epsilon_n$ we obtain that the event A_n implies

$$\sup_{t \in [t_{n-1}, t'_n)} |X(t) - X(t_{n-1})| \le a_n^{-1} |\xi_n - \xi_{n-1}| + C_\epsilon(\omega) \widetilde{\Delta}_{n-1}^{\alpha-\epsilon} + \epsilon_n.$$

Moreover, by Hölder continuity of $z(t)$ this implies that also

$$\sup_{t \in [t_{n-1}, t'_n)} |X(t) - X(t_{n-1})| \le C(\omega) a_n^{-1} \Delta_n + C_\epsilon(\omega) \widetilde{\Delta}_{n-1}^{\alpha-\epsilon} + \epsilon_n. \qquad (4.5)$$

Now the idea is to choose parameters such that (4.5) takes place only finite number of times. Next we will study the continuity of the integral. For this it suffices to show that $\int_{\tau_n}^{1} \psi(s) dX(s) \to 0$, $n \to \infty$, which would follow from $\|\psi\|_{\beta, [\tau_n, 1]} \to 0$, $n \to \infty$. Assume now that we have chosen parameters such that (4.5) takes place only finite number of times. We write

$$\|\psi\|_{\beta; [\tau_n, 1]} = I_1 + I_2,$$

where

$$I_1 = \int_{\tau_n}^{1} \frac{|\psi(t)|}{(t - \tau_n)^\beta} ds, \quad I_2 = \int_{\tau_n}^{1} \int_{\tau_n}^{t} \frac{|\psi(t) - \psi(s)|}{(t - s)^{\beta+1}} ds\, dt.$$

We follow arguments presented in Ref. 4 to obtain bounds for terms I_1 and I_2 with our general parameters, and some technical details will be omitted. First we estimate

$$I_1 = \int_{\tau_n}^{t_n} \frac{|\psi(t)|}{(t - \tau_n)^\beta} dt + \sum_{k=n}^{\infty} \int_{t_k}^{t_{k+1}} \frac{|\psi(t)|}{(t - \tau_n)^\beta} dt$$

$$\le C a_n \Delta_n^{1-\beta} + C \sum_{k=n}^{\infty} \frac{a_k \Delta_k}{(t_k - \tau_{n-1})^\beta} \le C \sum_{k=n}^{\infty} a_k \Delta_k^{1-\beta}.$$

For I_2 we write

$$I_2 = \sum_{k=n}^{\infty} \int_{t_k}^{\tau_{k+1}} \int_{\tau_n}^{t} \psi(t, s) ds\, dt + \sum_{k=n}^{\infty} \int_{\tau_k}^{t_k} \int_{\tau_n}^{t} \psi(t, s) ds\, dt$$

$$= \sum_{k=n}^{\infty} \int_{t_k}^{\tau_{k+1}} \int_{\tau_n}^{t_k} \psi(t, s) ds\, dt + \sum_{k=n}^{\infty} \int_{\tau_k}^{t_k} \int_{\tau_n}^{\tau_k} \psi(t, s) ds\, dt$$

$$+ \sum_{k=n}^{\infty} \int_{t_k}^{\tau_{k+1}} \int_{t_k}^{t} \psi(t,s) \mathrm{ds}\, \mathrm{dt} + \sum_{k=n}^{\infty} \int_{\tau_k}^{t_k} \int_{\tau_k}^{t} \psi(t,s) \mathrm{ds}\, \mathrm{dt}$$

$$=: J_1 + J_2 + J_3 + J_4,$$

where $\psi(t,s) = |\psi(t) - \psi(s)| (t-s)^{-\beta-1}$. Now arguments in Ref. 4 imply that we have

$$J_1 \leq C \sum_{k=n}^{\infty} a_k \Delta_k^{1-\beta},$$

$$J_2 \leq C \sum_{k=n}^{\infty} a_k \Delta_k^{1-\beta},$$

and

$$J_4 \leq C \sum_{k=n}^{\infty} \widetilde{\Delta}_k^{-1} \Delta_k^{2-\beta}.$$

Moreover, for J_3 we get by Hölder continuity of X that

$$J_3 \leq C(\omega) \sum_{k=n}^{\infty} a_k \epsilon_k^{-1} \Delta_k^{1+\alpha-\epsilon-\beta}.$$

To summarize, we need to choose parameters such that (4.5) happens only finite number of times and

(1)
$$\sum_{k=n}^{\infty} a_k \Delta_k^{1-\beta} \to 0,$$

(2)
$$\sum_{k=n}^{\infty} \widetilde{\Delta}_k^{-1} \Delta_k^{2-\beta} \to 0,$$

(3)
$$\sum_{k=n}^{\infty} a_k \epsilon_k^{-1} \Delta_k^{1+\alpha-\epsilon-\beta} \to 0.$$

Step 3. Analysis of the parameters. Next we prove that we can choose parameters such that we obtain (1) − (3) and (4.5) happens only finite number of times. For simplicity let us first put $a_n = \Delta_n^{-\mu}$, $\widetilde{\Delta}_n = \Delta_n^{\gamma}$, and $\epsilon_n = \Delta_n^{\kappa}$ for some parameters μ, γ and κ. With these choices (4.5) implies that

$$\sup_{t \in [t_{n-1}, t_n')} |X(t) - X(t_{n-1})| \leq C(\omega) \Delta_n^{\lambda},$$

where

$$\lambda = \min(\mu + a, \gamma(\alpha - \epsilon), \kappa).$$

Moreover, for any small number $\hat{\epsilon}$ there exists $N(\omega)$ such that

$$C(\omega)\Delta_n^{\hat{\epsilon}} \leq 1, \quad n \geq N(\omega).$$

Note now that the restriction $\epsilon \leq T^\alpha$ in Assumption 2 implies that we have to choose parameters such that $\Delta_n^{\lambda-\hat{\epsilon}} < \Delta_n^\alpha$, or equivalently $\lambda - \hat{\epsilon} > \alpha$. With such choices and applying Assumption 2 we obtain

$$\mathbb{P}\left(\sup_{t\in[t_{n-1},t_n')}|X(t) - X(t_{n-1})| \leq \Delta_n^{\lambda-\hat{\epsilon}}\right) \leq exp\left(-C\Delta_n^{1-\frac{\lambda-\hat{\epsilon}}{\alpha}}\right)$$

which is clearly summable provided Δ_n converges to zero fast enough.

Consider next restrictions $(1) - (3)$. With our choices we demand that

$$\sum_{k=n}^{\infty} \Delta_k^{1-\beta-\mu} \to 0,$$

$$\sum_{k=n}^{\infty} \Delta_k^{2-\beta-\gamma} \to 0,$$

and

$$\sum_{k=n}^{\infty} \Delta_k^{1+\alpha-\epsilon-\beta-\mu-\kappa} \to 0.$$

Again, these conditions are clearly satisfied provided that all the exponents are positive and Δ_k decays to zero fast enough. Hence, by collecting all restrictions, we obtain that we have to choose β, μ, κ, γ, ϵ, and $\hat{\epsilon}$ such that;

(1) $\mu + a - \hat{\epsilon} > \alpha$,
(2) $\kappa - \hat{\epsilon} > \alpha$,
(3) $\gamma(\alpha - \epsilon) - \hat{\epsilon} > \alpha$,
(4) $1 - \beta - \mu > 0$,
(5) $2 - \beta - \kappa > 0$,
(6) $1 + \alpha - \epsilon - \beta - \mu - \kappa > 0$.

The first three restrictions arises from Assumption 2 and the latter three from $(1) - (3)$. Note also that by choosing ϵ and $\hat{\epsilon}$ small enough we can actually omit them on the conditions $(1) - (6)$. Now (3) implies that $\gamma > 1$ which is consistent with $\widetilde{\Delta}_n \leq \Delta_n/2$ for n large enough. Next combining (4) and (1) we obtain that

$$\alpha - a < \mu < 1 - \beta$$

which is possible if we choose $\beta \in (1 - \alpha, 1 - \alpha + a)$. Next combining (2) and (5) we obtain

$$\alpha < \kappa < 2 - \beta,$$

and together with restrictions on β this is possible if

$$\alpha < \kappa < 1 + \alpha - a.$$

This is clearly possible since we can, without loss of generality, assume that $a < \alpha$. It remains to study (6). By choosing $\mu = \alpha - a + \delta$ and $\kappa = \alpha + \delta$ for δ small enough we obtain

$$1 + \alpha - \beta - \mu - \kappa = 1 + \alpha - \beta - \alpha + a - \delta - \alpha - \delta$$
$$= 1 - \beta + a - \alpha - 2\delta$$
$$> 0$$

since $\beta < 1 - \alpha + a$. To conclude, we obtained that we can choose parameters properly and it remains to choose Δ_n such that it converges to zero fast enough. $\qquad \square$

Remark 4.2. In Ref. 4 the authors defined $\Delta_n = n^{-\nu}$ and then chose ν properly to obtain the result. Now we obtained that one can choose Δ_n in many different ways. For example, one can choose $\Delta_n = \frac{K}{2^n}$ with $K = \left(\sum_{k=1}^{\infty} 2^{-k}\right)^{-1}$.

4.2. *Representation in the mixed case*

Next we turn to the representation w.r.t. the mixed fractional Brownian motion $B^H + W$ with $H \in (1/2, 1)$. We recall that the integral w.r.t. W is understood in the Itô sense, that w.r.t. B^H, in the generalized Lebesgue–Stieltjes sense.

Theorem 4.4. *Assume that the filtration $\mathbb{F}$ is left-continuous at 1. Then for any $\mathcal{F}_1$-measurable random variable ξ there exists an $\mathbb{F}$-adapted process ψ such that*

$$\int_0^1 \psi(t)\mathrm{d}(B^H(t) + W(t)) = \xi \qquad (4.6)$$

a.s.

Proof. The proof is similar to that of the main result in Ref. 1. Choose some $\beta \in (1 - H, 1/2)$. In view of the left-continuity of $\mathbb{F}$ at 1, for each k there exists an $\mathcal{F}_{1-2^{-k}}$-measurable random variable ξ_k such that $\xi_k \to \xi$, $k \to \infty$, a.s. Take a subsequence $k(n) \to \infty$, $n \to \infty$ such that

$$\mathbb{P}\left(\left|\xi_{k(n)} - \xi\right| > n^{-3}\right) \le n^{-2} \qquad (4.7)$$

and denote $t_n = 1 - 2^{-k(n)}$. The integrand ψ will be of the form $\psi = \sum_{n=1}^{\infty}(t_{n+1} - t)^{-1/2}\mathbf{1}_{[t_n, \tau_n)}$ with some $\tau_n \in (t_n, t_{n+1}]$. First we make some a priori estimates concerning the integrand. To this end, consider

$$\|\psi\|_{\beta;[t_n, t_{n+1}]} = I_1 + I_2,$$

where

$$I_1 = \int_{t_n}^{t_{n+1}} \frac{|\psi(t)|}{(t - t_n)^\beta}\mathrm{d}t = \int_0^{\tau_n} \frac{(t_{n+1} - t)^{-1/2}}{(t - t_n)^\beta}\mathrm{d}t \le C(t_{n+1} - t_n)^{1/2 - \beta};$$

$$I_2 = \int_{t_n}^{t_{n+1}} \int_{t_n}^t \frac{|\psi(t) - \psi(s)|}{(t - s)^{\beta+1}}\mathrm{d}s\,\mathrm{d}t$$

$$= \int_{t_n}^{\tau_n} \int_{t_n}^{t} \frac{\left| (t_{n+1} - t)^{-1/2} - (t_{n+1} - s)^{-1/2} \right|}{(t - s)^{\beta + 1}} \, ds \, dt$$

$$+ \int_{\tau_n}^{t_{n+1}} \int_0^{\tau_n} \frac{(t_{n+1} - s)^{-1/2}}{(t - s)^{\beta + 1}} \, ds \, dt$$

$$\leq \int_{t_n}^{\tau_n} \int_{t_n}^{t} \frac{ds \, dt}{(t_{n+1} - t)^{1/2} (t_{n+1} - s)^{1/2} (t - s)^{\beta + 1/2}}$$

$$+ C \int_0^{\tau_n} (t - \tau_n)^{-\beta - 1/2} dt \leq C(t_{n+1} - t_n)^{1/2 - \beta}.$$

In particular, denoting $v_n^H = \int_{t_n}^{t_{n+1}} \psi(t) dB^H(t)$, we have

$$\left| v_n^H \right| \leq C(t_{n+1} - t_n)^{1/2 - \beta} \Lambda(B^H), \tag{4.8}$$

whence

$$\mathbb{P}(\left| v_n^H \right| \geq n^{-3}) \leq \mathbb{P}\left(\left| \Lambda(B^H) \right| \geq C n^{-3} (t_{n+1} - t_n)^{\beta - 1/2} \right)$$

$$\leq \mathbb{P}\left(\left| \Lambda(B^H) \right| \geq C n^{-3} 2^{(1/2 - \beta)n} \right)$$

$$\leq C \mathbb{E} \left| \Lambda(B^H) \right| n^3 2^{(\beta - 1/2)n},$$

consequently,

$$\sum_{n=1}^{\infty} \mathbb{P}(\left| v_n^H \right| \geq n^{-3}) < \infty. \tag{4.9}$$

Now we define τ_n consecutively. Denote $v(t) = \int_0^t \psi(s) d(B^H(s) + W(s))$. For given $n \geq 1$ assume that τ_k is defined for $k = 1, \ldots, n-1$ (for $n = 0$, assume nothing) and denote $v_n^W(t) = \int_{t_n}^t (t_{n+1} - t)^{-1/2} dW(t)$. Since $\int_{t_n}^{t_{n+1}} (t_{n+1} - t) dt = +\infty$, we have $\liminf \int_{t_n}^t (t_{n+1} - t)^{-1/2} dW(s) = -\infty$ a.s., $\limsup \int_{t_n}^t (t_{n+1} - t)^{-1/2} dW(s) = +\infty$ a.s. Therefore, the stopping time $\tau_n = \inf\{t \geq t_n : v_n^W(t) = \xi_{k(n)} - v(t_n)\} \wedge t_{n+1}$ satisfies $\tau_n < t_{n+1}$ a.s.

We need to show (4.6). First we argue that $\int_0^1 \psi(t)^2 dt < \infty$ so that the integral $\int_0^1 \psi(s) dW(s)$ is well defined. Denote $G_n = \int_{t_n}^{t_{n+1}} \psi(t)^2 dt$. As in Ref. 1, we have $\mathbb{P}(G_n \geq n^{-2} \mid \mathcal{F}_{t_n}) \leq n \left| \xi_{k(n)} - v(t_n) \right|$. For $n \geq 2$, note that

$$v(t_n) = v(t_{n-1}) + \int_{t_{n-1}}^{t_n} \psi(t) dW(t) + \int_{t_{n-1}}^{t_n} \psi(t) dB^H(t)$$

$$= \xi_{k(n-1)} + \int_{t_{n-1}}^{t_n} \psi(t) dB^H(t) = \xi_{k(n-1)} + v_n^H \tag{4.10}$$

and estimate

$$\left| \xi_{k(n)} - v(t_n) \right| \leq \left| \xi_{k(n)} - \xi \right| + \left| \xi_{k(n-1)} - \xi \right| + \left| v_n^H \right|.$$

Therefore, taking into account (4.7) and (4.9), we get that

$$\sum_{n=1}^{\infty} \mathbb{P}(G_n \geq n^{-2}) \leq \sum_{n=1}^{\infty} \left(3n^{-2} + \mathbb{P}(n \left| \xi_{k(n)} - v(t_n) \right| \geq 3n^{-2}) \right)$$

$$\leq \sum_{n=1}^{\infty} \left(3n^{-2} + \mathbb{P}(\left| \xi_{k(n)} - \xi \right| \geq n^{-3}) \right.$$

$$\left. + \mathbb{P}(\left| \xi_{k(n-1)} - \xi \right| \geq n^{-3}) + \mathbb{P}\left(\left| v_n^H \right| \geq n^{-3} \right) \right) < \infty.$$

Then the Borel–Cantelli lemma implies that $\int_0^1 \psi(t)^2 dt = \sum_{n=1}^{\infty} G_n < \infty$ a.s.

To show the existence of the integral $\int_0^1 \psi(t) dB^H(t)$, we write $\|\psi\|_{\beta;[0,1]} \leq \sum_{n=1}^{\infty} \|\psi\|_{\beta;[t_n,t_{n+1}]}$ and use the above estimates for $\|\psi\|_{\beta;[t_n,t_{n+1}]}$.

In view of (4.8) and (4.10), $v(t_n) \to \xi$, $n \to \infty$. It remains to prove that $v(1) - v(t_n) = \int_{t_n}^1 \psi(t) d(B^H(t)+W(s)) \to 0$, $n \to \infty$. The convergence $\int_{t_n}^1 \psi(t) dW(t) \to 0$, $n \to \infty$ follows from the convergence of the series $\sum_{n=1}^{\infty} G_n$, and $\left| \int_{t_n}^1 \psi(t) dB^H(t) \right| \leq \sum_{k=n}^{\infty} \left| v_n^H \right| < \infty$ thanks to (4.8), which concludes the proof. $\qquad\square$

Remark 4.3. It is straightforward to generalize the statement to the case where $X(t) = \int_0^t \sigma(s) dW(s) + Z(t)$, where the process σ is an $\mathbb{F}$-adapted bounded non-vanishing process, and Z is Hölder continuous of some order $\alpha > 1/2$.

Acknowledgments

The first author would like to thank Dr. Maria Victoria Carpio-Bernido and Dr. Christopher Bernido for their great hospitality during his visit to Jagna in January 2014.

References

1. R. M. Dudley, Wiener functionals as Ito integrals, *Ann. Probab.* **5**, 140 (1977).
2. Y. Mishura, G. Shevchenko and E. Valkeila, Random variables as pathwise integrals with respect to fractional Brownian motion, *Stochastic Process. Appl.* **123**, 2353 (2013).
3. L. Viitasaari, Integral representation of random variables with respect to gaussian processes (2013), arXiv:math.PR/1307.7559.
4. G. Shevchenko and L. Viitasaari, Integral representation with adapted continuous integrand with respect to fractional Brownian motion (2014), arXiv:math.PR/1403.2066.
5. M. Zähle, Integration with respect to fractal functions and stochastic calculus. I, *Probab. Theory Relat. Fields* **111**, 333 (1998).

7th Jagna International Workshop (2014)
International Journal of Modern Physics: Conference Series
Vol. 36 (2015) 1560005 (11 pages)
© The Author
DOI: 10.1142/S2010194515600058

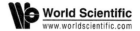

A white noise analysis of Volterra processes

H. P. Suryawan

Department of Mathematics, Sanata Dharma University,
Yogyakarta, Indonesia
herrypribs@usd.ac.id

Published 2 January 2015

In this paper we present a realization of Volterra processes within the white noise analysis framework. We show that Donsker's delta functions of Volterra processes are elements from the space of Hida distributions. An explicit expression for the corresponding chaos decomposition in terms of Wick tensor powers of white noise is also given.

Keywords: Volterra processes; white noise analysis; Volterra white noise.

1. Introduction

There has been a growing interest in the study of Volterra processes, i.e. Gaussian processes having representation as the stochastic integral of a time dependent kernel with respect to the standard Brownian motion. The main motivation comes from the diverse applications in the fields of telecommunications and internet traffic, turbulence in liquids, image analysis and synthesis, geophysics, and mathematical finance, to name just a few. The class of Volterra processes includes Brownian bridge, Ornstein-Uhlenbeck process, and fractional Brownian motion. Several works on the Volterra process, the corresponding stochastic calculus, and their applications can be found in Refs. 2, 3, 5 and 9.

Let us denote by I an index set which will be a compact interval $[0, T]$, $0 < T < \infty$, the nonnegative half line $[0, \infty)$ or the real line $\mathbb{R}$. Given a locally square-integrable kernel K, i.e. a mapping $K : I \times I \to \mathbb{R}$ such that $K \in L^2_{\mathrm{loc}}(I^2)$. It is well-known that K induces a Hilbert-Schmidt operator $\mathcal{K} : L^2(I) \to L^2(I)$ in the following way: an element $f \in L^2(I)$ is mapped to the mapping $t \mapsto \int_I K(t, s) f(s)\, ds$. We assume the following conditions:

(i) K is a Volterra kernel, i.e. $K(0, s) = 0$ for all $s \in I$ and $K(t, s) = 0$ for $s > t$.

(ii) The family $\{K(t, \cdot) : t \in I\}$ is linearly independent.

(iii) There are positive constants C and α such that for all $t, s \in I$

$$\int_I |K(t, r) - K(s, r)|^2 \, dr \leq C \, |t - s|^\alpha .$$

A stochastic process $X = (X_t)_{t \in I}$ defined on a complete probability space $(\Omega, \mathcal{F}, \mathbb{P})$ admitting a representation

$$X_t = \int_I K(t, r) \, dB_r, \tag{1}$$

where $B = (B_t)_{t \in I}$ denotes standard Brownian motion on $(\Omega, \mathcal{F}, \mathbb{P})$ and K is a kernel satisfying conditions (i)-(iii) is called a *Volterra process*. Assumption (i) implies that X is adapted to the natural filtration of the Brownian motion B. From (iii) we know that $K(t, \cdot) \in L^2(I)$ for each $t \in I$ and hence, the process X is well-defined as a family of Wiener integrals. Condition (iii) also guarantees the existence of a Hölder continuous modification of the process X. It is clear that X is a centered Gaussian process with covariance structure

$$\operatorname{cov}(X_t, X_s) = \int_I K(t, r) K(s, r) \, dr, \quad t, s \in I.$$

Note that the assumption (ii) guarantees that the covariance function is indeed positive semidefinite on I. Informally, we can consider (1) as a generalized stochastic Volterra integral equation with solution white noise $\dot{B}_t = \frac{d}{dt} B_t$.

Since with probability one Brownian motion is nowhere differentiable, the commonly used term white noise $\dot{B}_t$ must be treated carefully. A branch of stochastic analysis which deals with the rigorous study of the white noise is known as white noise analysis. It was first introduced by T. Hida in 1976. The basic idea is to do a stochastic analysis where the underlying random variable is not Brownian motion but rather its velocity, white noise. Being independent at each time, white noise provides a suitable infinite dimensional coordinate system. Due to the Gaussian structure it is natural to study the class of Volterra processes within the framework of white noise analysis. It is our main goal to build a comprehensive study of the white noise approach to Volterra processes and to develop some applications. In this paper we present some preliminary results. We remark that the study of Volterra process by using white noise theory has been initiated in the work of Nualart.[9] There the author focused on the stochastic integration with respect to fractional Brownian motion using Malliavin calculus as well as white noise analysis.

The present paper is organized as follows. Section 2 contains a summary on some standard facts from the theory of white noise analysis. In Section 3 we present a realization of Volterra processes on the white noise space. We also prove that the Donsker delta function of a Volterra process exists as a Hida distribution. As a corollary we provide an explicit expression for the corresponding chaos decomposition. Conclusions and future works are given in Section 4.

2. Basics of White Noise Analysis

In order to make the paper self-contained, we summarize some fundamental concepts of white noise analysis used throughout this paper. For a more comprehensive explanation including various applications of white noise theory, see for example the books of Hida et al,[4] Kuo[7] and Obata.[10] Let $(\mathcal{S}'_d(\mathbb{R}), \mathcal{C}, \mu)$ be the $\mathbb{R}^d$-valued white noise space, i.e., $\mathcal{S}'_d(\mathbb{R})$ is the space of $\mathbb{R}^d$-valued tempered distributions, $\mathcal{C}$ is the Borel σ-algebra generated by cylinder sets on $\mathcal{S}'_d(\mathbb{R})$, and the white noise probability measure μ is uniquely determined through the Bochner-Minlos theorem by fixing the characteristic function

$$C(\vec{f}) := \int_{\mathcal{S}'_d(\mathbb{R})} \exp\left(i\langle \vec{\omega}, \vec{f}\rangle\right) d\mu(\vec{\omega}) = \exp\left(-\frac{1}{2}|\vec{f}|_0^2\right)$$

for all $\mathbb{R}^d$-valued Schwartz test function $\vec{f} \in \mathcal{S}_d(\mathbb{R})$. Here $|\cdot|_0$ denotes the usual norm in the real Hilbert space of all $\mathbb{R}^d$-valued Lebesgue square-integrable functions $L^2_d(\mathbb{R})$ and $\langle \cdot, \cdot \rangle$ denotes the dual pairing between $\mathcal{S}'_d(\mathbb{R})$ and $\mathcal{S}_d(\mathbb{R})$. The dual pairing is considered as the bilinear extension of the inner product on $L^2_d(\mathbb{R})$, i.e. $\langle \vec{g}, \vec{f}\rangle = \sum_{j=1}^d \int_{\mathbb{R}} g_j(x) f_j(x)\, dx$ for all $\vec{g} = (g_1, \ldots, g_d) \in L^2_d(\mathbb{R})$ and $\vec{f} = (f_1, \ldots, f_d) \in \mathcal{S}_d(\mathbb{R})$. We have also the Gel'fand triple, i.e. the continuous and dense embeddings of spaces $\mathcal{S}_d(\mathbb{R}) \hookrightarrow L^2_d(\mathbb{R}) \hookrightarrow \mathcal{S}'_d(\mathbb{R})$. We choose the family of the Hilbertian norms which topologizes $\mathcal{S}_d(\mathbb{R})$ as the one generated by the Hamiltonian operator of a harmonic oscillator $H = -\frac{d^2}{dx^2} + (x^2 + 1)$ (acting in each component) as $\left|\vec{f}\right|_p^2 = \left|H^p\vec{f}\right|_0^2 = \sum_{j=1}^d \sum_{n=0}^\infty (2n+2)^{2p}(f_j, e_n)^2$ where e_n, $n \geq 0$ denotes the n-th Hermite function.

Recall that the complex Hilbert space $L^2(\mu) := L^2(\mathcal{S}'_d(\mathbb{R}), \mathcal{C}, \mu; \mathbb{C})$ is canonically unitary isomorphic to the d-fold tensor product of Fock space of symmetric square-integrable function, i.e. $L^2(\mu) \cong \left(\bigoplus_{k=0}^\infty L^2_s(\mathbb{R}^k, k! d^k x)\right)^{\otimes d}$ via the so-called Wiener-Itô-Segal isomorphism. Thus, we have the unique chaos decomposition of an element $F \in L^2(\mu)$,

$$F(\omega_1, \ldots, \omega_d) = \sum_{(m_1,\ldots,m_d) \in \mathbb{N}_0^d} \left\langle :\omega_1^{\otimes m_1}: \otimes \ldots \otimes :\omega_d^{\otimes m_d}:, \vec{f}_{(m_1,\ldots,m_d)}\right\rangle, \qquad (2)$$

with kernel functions $\vec{f}_{(m_1,\ldots,m_d)}$ of the m-th chaos are in the Fock space. Here $:\omega_j^{\otimes m_j}:$ denotes the m_j-th Wick tensor power of $\omega_j \in \mathcal{S}'_1(\mathbb{R})$. We also introduce the following notations

$$\mathbf{m} = (m_1, \ldots, m_d) \in \mathbb{N}_0^d, \quad m = \sum_{j=1}^d m_j, \quad \mathbf{m}! = \prod_{j=1}^d m_j!,$$

which simplify (2) to $F(\vec{\omega}) = \sum_{\mathbf{m} \in \mathbb{N}_0^d} \left\langle :\vec{\omega}^{\otimes \mathbf{m}}:, \vec{f}_{\mathbf{m}}\right\rangle$, $\vec{\omega} \in \mathcal{S}'_d(\mathbb{R})$. Using, for example, the Wiener-Itô chaos decomposition theorem (2) and the second quantization operator of H we can construct the Gel'fand triple $(\mathcal{S}) \hookrightarrow L^2(\mu) \hookrightarrow (\mathcal{S})^*$. Here $(\mathcal{S})$ is the space of white noise test functions obtained by taking the intersection of a family of Hilbert subspaces of $L^2(\mu)$. It is equipped with the projective limit topology and has the structure of nuclear Frechet space. The space of white noise distributions $(\mathcal{S})^*$ is defined as the topological dual space of $(\mathcal{S})$. Elements of $(\mathcal{S})$ and $(\mathcal{S})^*$ are also known as *Hida test functions* and *Hida distributions*, respectively.

The *S-transform* of an element $\Phi \in (\mathcal{S})^*$ is defined as

$$(S\Phi)(\vec{f}) := \left\langle\!\left\langle \Phi, : \exp\left(\left\langle \cdot, \vec{f} \right\rangle\right) : \right\rangle\!\right\rangle, \quad \vec{f} \in \mathcal{S}_d(\mathbb{R}),$$

where

$$: \exp\left(\left\langle \cdot, \vec{f} \right\rangle\right) := \sum_{\mathbf{m} \in \mathbb{N}_0^d} \left\langle : \cdot^{\otimes \mathbf{m}} :, \vec{f}^{\otimes \mathbf{m}} \right\rangle = C(\vec{f}) \exp\left(\left\langle \cdot, \vec{f} \right\rangle\right),$$

is the so-called Wick exponential and $\langle\!\langle \cdot, \cdot \rangle\!\rangle$ denotes the dual pairing between $(\mathcal{S})^*$ and $(\mathcal{S})$. We define this dual pairing as the bilinear extension of the sesquilinear inner product on $L^2(\mu)$. The decomposition $S\Phi(\vec{f}) = \sum_{\mathbf{m} \in \mathbb{N}_0^d} \left\langle F_{\mathbf{m}}, \vec{f}^{\otimes \mathbf{m}} \right\rangle$ extends the chaos decomposition to $\Phi \in (\mathcal{S})^*$ with distribution-valued kernels $F_{\mathbf{m}}$ such that $\langle\!\langle \Phi, \varphi \rangle\!\rangle = \sum_{\mathbf{m} \in \mathbb{N}_0^d} \mathbf{m}! \langle F_{\mathbf{m}}, \vec{\varphi}_{\mathbf{m}} \rangle$, for every Hida test function $\varphi \in (\mathcal{S})$ with kernel functions $\vec{\varphi}_{\mathbf{m}}$. The S-transform provides a very useful way to deal with the Bochner integration of a family of Hida distributions which depend on an additional parameter. The following result is a corollary from the famous Potthoff-Streit characterization theorem, for details and proof see Ref. 6.

Theorem 2.1. *Let $(\Omega, \mathcal{A}, \nu)$ be a measure space and $\lambda \mapsto \Phi_\lambda$ be a mapping from Ω to $(\mathcal{S})^*$. If the S-transform of Φ_λ fulfills the following two conditions:*

(1) *the mapping $\lambda \mapsto S(\Phi_\lambda)(\vec{f})$ is measurable for all $\vec{f} \in \mathcal{S}_d(\mathbb{R})$, and*
(2) *there exist $C_1(\lambda) \in L^1(\Omega, \mathcal{A}, \nu)$, $C_2(\lambda) \in L^\infty(\Omega, \mathcal{A}, \nu)$ and a continuous quadratic form B on $\mathcal{S}_d(\mathbb{R})$ such that for all $z \in \mathbb{C}, \vec{f} \in \mathcal{S}_d(\mathbb{R})$*

$$\left| S(\Phi_\lambda)(z\vec{f}) \right| \le C_1(\lambda) \exp\left(C_2(\lambda)|z|^2 B(\vec{f}) \right),$$

then Φ_λ is Bochner integrable with respect to some Hilbertian norm which topologizing $(\mathcal{S})^*$. Hence $\int_\Omega \Phi_\lambda \, d\nu(\lambda) \in (\mathcal{S})^*$, and furthermore

$$S\left(\int_\Omega \Phi_\lambda \, d\nu(\lambda) \right) = \int_\Omega S(\Phi_\lambda) \, d\nu(\lambda).$$

3. Volterra Processes via White Noise Analysis

Let $K(t, -)$ be a Volterra kernel satisfying (i)–(iii). By using the general theory, see e.g. Refs. 4 and 10, we have that the real-valued random variable $X_t := \langle \cdot, K(t, -) \rangle$ defined on the white noise space is normally distributed with mean $\mathbb{E}_\mu(X_t) = \int_{\mathcal{S}'(\mathbb{R})} \langle \omega, K(t, -) \rangle \, d\mu(\omega) = 0$ and variance $\text{var}(X_t) = \int_{\mathcal{S}'(\mathbb{R})} |\langle \omega, K(t, -) \rangle|^2 \, d\mu(\omega) = \int_{\mathbb{R}} |K(t, s)|^2 \, ds$. Here $\mathbb{E}_\mu$ denotes the expectation with respect to the white noise measure μ. As a consequence, the finite dimensional distributions of stochastic process $(X_t)_{t \in I}$ coincide with those of Volterra process. Hence, the following representation of Volterra process on the white noise space is well-defined.

Definition 3.1. Let $K, K_1, \ldots, K_d$ be kernels satisfying assumptions (i)-(iii). A centered Gaussian process $X = (X_t)_{t \in I}$ defined on the white noise space by $X_t := \langle \cdot, K(t, -) \rangle$ is called a (one-dimensional) Volterra process. A d-dimensional Volterra process $X = (X_t)_{t \in I}$ is given by the vector $X_t = (\langle \cdot, K_1(t, -) \rangle, \ldots, \langle \cdot, K_d(t, -) \rangle)$, where $(\langle \cdot, K_1(t, -) \rangle)_{t \in I}, \ldots, (\langle \cdot, K_d(t, -) \rangle)_{t \in I}$ are d independent one-dimensional Volterra processes.

The notation $\langle \cdot, K(t, -) \rangle$ has the following meaning. The $\cdot$ indicates a tempered distribution $\omega \in \mathcal{S}'(\mathbb{R})$ in the variable $-$. Thus, $\langle \omega(s), K(t, s) \rangle$ only depends on the parameter t. Moreover, for a fixed $\omega \in \mathcal{S}'(\mathbb{R})$, it represents a sample path of the stochastic process X. Note that we have to take $\vec{\omega} = (\omega_1, \ldots, \omega_d) \in \mathcal{S}'_d(\mathbb{R})$ as a vector of d independent white noises to ensure the independence of d Volterra processes in the multidimensional case. Recall that we define Volterra process on white noise space up to finite dimensional distributions. The assumption (iii) implies the existence of a Hölder continuous modification of the process X. Indeed, let $p \in [1, \infty)$, then there exists a constant c_p such that for each $t, s \in I$:

$$
\begin{aligned}
\mathbb{E}_\mu \left(|X_t - X_s|^p \right) &= \mathbb{E}_\mu \left(|\langle \cdot, K(t, -) \rangle - \langle \cdot, K(s, -) \rangle|^p \right) \\
&\leq \left(\mathbb{E}_\mu \left(|\langle \cdot, K(t, -) - K(s, -) \rangle|^2 \right) \right)^{p/2} \\
&\leq c_p \left(\int_I |K(t, r) - K(s, r)|^2 \, dr \right)^{p/2} \\
&\leq c_p \, |t - s|^{\beta p/2} \\
&\leq c_p \, |t - s|^{1+\eta},
\end{aligned}
$$

for some $\eta > 0$ and $p > \beta/2$. Hence, according to the Kolmogorov-Chentsov continuity theorem X has a modification with sample paths which are Hölder continuous of index γ for every $\gamma < \beta/2$.

In several applications, such as in the context of Feynman path integral and Edwards' polymer model, we need to "pin" a Volterra process at some point $c \in \mathbb{R}^d$. For this purpose we consider *Donsker's delta function* of a Volterra process. It is defined as the informal composition of the Dirac delta function $\delta_d \in \mathcal{S}'(\mathbb{R}^d)$ with a d-dimensional Volterra process $(X_t)_{t \in [0,T]}$, i.e., $\delta_d (X_t - c)$. We can give a precise meaning to Donsker's delta function as a Hida distribution.

Theorem 3.1. *Let I an index set which is either a compact interval $[0, T]$, $0 < T < \infty$, the nonnegative half line $[0, \infty)$ or the real line $\mathbb{R}$. For a d-dimensional Volterra process*

$$
X = (X_t)_{t \in I} = \left(\left\langle \cdot, \vec{K}(t, -) \right\rangle \right)_{t \in I} = (\langle \cdot, K_1(t, -) \rangle, \ldots, \langle \cdot, K_d(t, -) \rangle)_{t \in I}
$$

and $c = (c_1, \ldots, c_d) \in \mathbb{R}^d$, the Bochner integral

$$\delta\left(\left\langle\cdot,\vec{K}(t,-)\right\rangle - c\right) := \left(\frac{1}{2\pi}\right)^d \int_{\mathbb{R}^d} \exp\left(i\lambda\left(\left\langle\cdot,\vec{K}(t,-)\right\rangle - c\right)\right) d\lambda$$

is a Hida distribution with S-transform given by

$$S\delta\left(\left\langle\cdot,\vec{K}(t,-)\right\rangle - c\right)\left(\vec{f}\right)$$

$$= \left(\frac{1}{2\pi}\right)^{d/2}\left(\prod_{j=1}^{d}\frac{1}{|K_j(t,-)|_0}\right)\exp\left(-\frac{1}{2}\sum_{j=1}^{d}\frac{(\langle f_j, K_j(t,-)\rangle - c_j)^2}{|K_j(t,-)|_0^2}\right)$$

for all $\vec{f} \in \mathcal{S}_d(\mathbb{R})$.

Proof. We are going to show that

$$\int_{\mathbb{R}^d} \exp\left(i\lambda\left(\left\langle\cdot,\vec{K}(t,-)\right\rangle - c\right)\right) d\lambda \in (\mathcal{S})^*.$$

First of all we fix the following notations: $\lambda\vec{K}(t,-) := \sum_{j=1}^{d}\lambda_j K_j(t,-)$, $\lambda\left\langle\vec{f},\vec{K}(t,-)\right\rangle = \left\langle\vec{f},\lambda\vec{K}(t,-)\right\rangle := \sum_{j=1}^{d}\lambda_j f_j K_j(t,-)$, and $|\lambda|^2\left|\vec{K}(t,-)\right|_0^2 := \sum_{j=1}^{d}\lambda_j^2|K_j(t,-)|_0^2$. Let $F_\lambda(\vec{f}) := S\exp\left(i\lambda\left(\left\langle\cdot,\vec{K}(t,-)\right\rangle - c\right)\right)(\vec{f})$, $\vec{f} \in \mathcal{S}_d(\mathbb{R})$. Hence

$$F_\lambda(\vec{f}) = \left\langle\!\left\langle\exp\left(i\lambda\left(\left\langle\cdot,\vec{K}(t,-)\right\rangle - c\right)\right),:\exp\left(\left\langle\cdot,\vec{f}\right\rangle\right):\right\rangle\!\right\rangle$$

$$= \int_{\mathcal{S}_d'(\mathbb{R})} \exp\left(i\lambda\left(\left\langle\vec{\omega},\vec{K}(t,-)\right\rangle - c\right)\right)\exp\left(-\frac{1}{2}|\vec{f}|_0^2\right)\exp\left(\left\langle\vec{\omega},\vec{f}\right\rangle\right) d\mu(\vec{\omega})$$

$$= \exp\left(-\frac{1}{2}|\vec{f}|_0^2\right)\int_{\mathcal{S}_d'(\mathbb{R})} \exp\left(-i\lambda c\right)\exp\left(\left\langle\vec{\omega},i\lambda\vec{K}(t,-)+\vec{f}\right\rangle\right) d\mu(\vec{\omega})$$

$$= \exp\left(-\frac{1}{2}|\vec{f}|_0^2\right)\exp\left(-i\lambda c\right)\exp\left(\frac{1}{2}\left|\vec{f}+i\lambda\vec{K}(t,-)\right|_0^2\right)$$

$$= \exp\left(-\frac{1}{2}|\vec{f}|_0^2\right)\exp\left(-i\lambda c\right)\exp\left(\frac{1}{2}|\vec{f}|_0^2\right)\exp\left(i\lambda\left\langle\vec{f},\vec{K}(t,-)\right\rangle\right)$$

$$\times \exp\left(-\frac{1}{2}|\lambda|^2\left|\vec{K}(t,-)\right|_0^2\right)$$

$$= \exp\left(-\frac{1}{2}|\lambda|^2\left|\vec{K}(t,-)\right|_0^2\right)\exp\left(i\lambda\left(\left\langle\vec{f},\vec{K}(t,-)\right\rangle - c\right)\right).$$

The mapping $\lambda \mapsto F_\lambda(\vec{f})$ is continuous for all $\vec{f} \in \mathcal{S}_d(\mathbb{R})$. Thus, the measurability with respect to Lebesgue measure λ is fulfilled. Furthermore, for $z \in \mathbb{C}$, $\vec{f} \in \mathcal{S}_d(\mathbb{R})$:

$$\left| F_\lambda(z\vec{f}) \right|$$

$$\leq \exp\left(-\frac{1}{2}|\lambda|^2 \left| \vec{K}(t,-) \right|_0^2 \right) \exp\left(|z| \left| \left\langle \vec{f}, \lambda \vec{K}(t,-) \right\rangle \right| \right)$$

$$= \exp\left(-\frac{1}{4}|\lambda|^2 |\vec{K}(t,-)|_0^2 \right)$$

$$\times \exp\left(-\left(\frac{1}{2}\left(|\lambda|^2 \left| \vec{K}(t,-) \right|_0^2 \right)^{1/2} - \frac{|z| \left| \left\langle \vec{f}, \lambda \vec{K}(t,-) \right\rangle \right|}{\left(|\lambda|^2 \left| \vec{K}(t,-) \right|_0^2 \right)^{1/2}} \right)^2 + \frac{|z|^2 \left| \left\langle \vec{f}, \lambda \vec{K}(t,-) \right\rangle \right|^2}{|\lambda|^2 \left| \vec{K}(t,-) \right|_0^2} \right)$$

$$\leq \exp\left(-\frac{1}{4}|\lambda|^2 \left| \vec{K}(t,-) \right|_0^2 \right) \exp\left(\frac{|z|^2}{|\lambda|^2 \left| \vec{K}(t,-) \right|_0^2} \left(\sum_{j=1}^d |\langle f_j, \lambda_j K_j(t,-)\rangle| \right)^2 \right)$$

$$\leq \exp\left(-\frac{1}{4}|\lambda|^2 \left| \vec{K}(t,-) \right|_0^2 \right) \exp\left(\frac{|z|^2}{|\lambda|^2 \left| \vec{K}(t,-) \right|_0^2} \left(\sum_{j=1}^d |f_j|_0 |\lambda_j K_j(t,-)|_0 \right)^2 \right)$$

$$\leq \exp\left(-\frac{1}{4} \sum_{j=1}^d \lambda_j^2 |K_j(t,-)|_0^2 \right)$$

$$\times \exp\left(\frac{|z|^2}{|\lambda|^2 \left| \vec{K}(t,-) \right|_0^2} \left(\sum_{j=1}^d |f_j|_0^2 \right) \left(\sum_{j=1}^d \lambda_j^2 |K_j(t,-)|_0^2 \right) \right)$$

$$= \exp\left(-\frac{1}{4}|\lambda|^2 \left| \vec{K}(t,-) \right|_0^2 \right) \exp\left(|z|^2 |\vec{f}|_0^2 \right).$$

The first factor is an integrable function of λ, and in the second exponential the factor is independent of λ. Hence, according to Theorem 2.1

$$\delta\left(\left\langle \cdot, \vec{K}(t,-) \right\rangle - c \right) \in (\mathcal{S})^*.$$

To obtain the S-transform of $\delta\left(\left\langle \cdot, \vec{K}(t,-) \right\rangle - c \right)$, we integrate $F_\lambda(\vec{f})$ over $\mathbb{R}^d$:

$$S\delta\left(\left\langle \cdot, \vec{K}(t,-) \right\rangle - c \right)(\vec{f})$$

$$= S\left(\left(\frac{1}{2\pi} \right)^d \int_{\mathbb{R}^d} \exp\left(i\lambda \left(\left\langle \cdot, \vec{K}(t,-) \right\rangle - c \right) \right) d\lambda \right)(\vec{f})$$

$$= \left(\frac{1}{2\pi}\right)^d \int_{\mathbb{R}^d} S \exp\left(i\left(\left\langle\cdot, \lambda\vec{K}(t,-)\right\rangle - c\right)\right) (\vec{f})\, d\lambda$$

$$= \left(\frac{1}{2\pi}\right)^d \int_{\mathbb{R}^d} \exp\left(-\frac{1}{2}|\lambda|^2 \left|\vec{K}(t,-)\right|_0^2\right) \exp\left(i\lambda\left(\left\langle\vec{f}, \vec{K}(t,-)\right\rangle - c\right)\right) d\lambda$$

$$= \left(\frac{1}{2\pi}\right)^d \prod_{j=1}^d \int_{\mathbb{R}} \exp\left(-\frac{1}{2}|K_j(t,-)|_0^2\lambda_j^2 + i\lambda_j\left(\langle f_j, K_j(t,-)\rangle - c_j\right)\right) d\lambda_j$$

$$= \left(\frac{1}{2\pi}\right)^d \prod_{j=1}^d \frac{\sqrt{\pi}}{\sqrt{\frac{1}{2}|K_j(t,-)|_0^2}} \exp\left(\frac{(i\left(\langle f_j, K_j(t,-)\rangle - c_j\right))^2}{2|K_j(t,-)|_0^2}\right)$$

$$= \left(\frac{1}{2\pi}\right)^{d/2} \left(\prod_{j=1}^d \frac{1}{|K_j(t,-)|_0}\right) \exp\left(-\frac{1}{2}\sum_{j=1}^d \frac{(\langle f_j, K_j(t,-)\rangle - c_j)^2}{|K_j(t,-)|_0^2}\right). \qquad \square$$

As an immediate consequence of Theorem 3.1 we obtain the generalized expectation of the Donsker delta function of a Volterra process

$$\mathbb{E}_\mu\left(\delta\left(\left\langle\cdot, \vec{K}(t,-)\right\rangle - c\right)\right) = \left(\frac{1}{2\pi}\right)^{d/2} \prod_{j=1}^d \frac{1}{|K_j(t,-)|_0} \exp\left(-\frac{1}{2}\left(\frac{c_j}{|K_j(t,-)|_0}\right)^2\right).$$

Moreover, from Theorem 3.1 we are able to derive the chaos decomposition for the Donsker delta function of Volterra process. In order to avoid complicated notations we present the result in the case $c = 0$.

Corollary 3.1. *Let $X = (X_t)_{t\in I}$ be a d-dimensional Volterra process. The kernel functions $F_{2\mathbf{m}}$ of $\delta\left(\left\langle\cdot, \vec{K}(t,-)\right\rangle\right)$ are given by*

$$F_{2\mathbf{m}}(u_1, \ldots, u_{2m}) = \left(-\frac{1}{2}\right)^m \left(\frac{1}{2\pi}\right)^{d/2} \frac{1}{\mathbf{m}!} \prod_{j=1}^d \frac{1}{|K_j(t,-)|_0^{1+2m_j}} \prod_{l=1}^{2m} K_j(t, u_l),$$

for each $\mathbf{m} \in \mathbb{N}_0^d$. All other odd kernel functions $F_{\mathbf{m}}$ vanish.

Some examples of Volterra processes, their realization on the white noise space together with their Donsker's delta functions are now in order.

(1) ***Brownian bridge***: Let $I = [0, T]$ and

$$K_j(t, s) = \mathbf{1}_{[0,t)}(s) - \frac{t}{T}\mathbf{1}_{[0,T)}(s), \quad j = 1, \ldots, d.$$

Then K_j satisfies assumptions (i)-(iii) and the stochastic process $(X_t)_{t\geq 0}$ with $X_t := \left\langle\cdot, \mathbf{1}_{[0,t)} - \frac{t}{T}\mathbf{1}_{[0,T)}\right\rangle$ is a d-dimensional Brownian bridge with length T starting in 0 at time 0 and ending in 0 at time T. Thus, we have the Bochner integral

$$\delta\left(\left\langle\cdot,\mathbf{1}_{[0,t)}-\frac{t}{T}\mathbf{1}_{[0,T)}\right\rangle-c\right)$$

$$:=\left(\frac{1}{2\pi}\right)^d\int_{\mathbb{R}^d}\exp\left(i\lambda\left(\left\langle\cdot,\mathbf{1}_{[0,t)}-\frac{t}{T}\mathbf{1}_{[0,T)}\right\rangle-c\right)\right)\,d\lambda$$

is a Hida distribution with S-transform given by

$$S\delta\left(\left\langle\cdot,\mathbf{1}_{[0,t)}-\frac{t}{T}\mathbf{1}_{[0,T)}\right\rangle-c\right)(\vec{f})$$

$$=\left(\frac{1}{\sqrt{2\pi\left(t-\frac{t^2}{T}\right)}}\right)^d$$

$$\times\exp\left(-\frac{1}{2\left(t-\frac{t^2}{T}\right)}\sum_{j=1}^d\left(\int_0^t f_j(x)\,dx-\frac{t}{T}\int_0^T f_j(x)\,dx-c_j\right)^2\right)$$

for all $\vec{f}\in\mathcal{S}_d(\mathbb{R})$.

(2) **Fractional Brownian motion**: Let $H\in(0,1)$, $I=[0,T]$, and

$$K_j(t,s)=\frac{(t-s)^{H-\frac{1}{2}}}{\sqrt{V_H}\Gamma(H+\frac{1}{2})}\,{}_1F_2\left(H-\frac{1}{2},\frac{1}{2}-H,H+\frac{1}{2},1-\frac{t}{s}\right)\mathbf{1}_{[0,t)}(s),$$

where ${}_1F_2$ is the Gauss hypergeometric function and $V_H=\frac{\Gamma(2-2H)\cos(\pi H)}{\pi H(1-2H)}$ is a normalizing constant which makes $\mathrm{var}(X_1)=1$. Then K_j satisfies assumptions (i)-(iii) and the stochastic process $\left(B_t^H\right)_{t\geq0}$ with $B_t^H:=\langle\cdot,K_j(t,-)\rangle$ is a d-dimensional fractional Brownian motion with Hurst parameter H, see e.g. Refs. 3 and 5. We can also define the fractional Brownian motion on the whole real line using the so-called moving average representation, i.e. $B_t^H:=\langle\cdot,K_j(t,-)\rangle$ where $K_j(t,s)=\frac{1}{C_H}\left((t-s)_+^{H-\frac{1}{2}}-(-s)_+^{H-\frac{1}{2}}\right)$ where $u_+=\max\{u,0\}$ and

$$C_H=\left(\int_0^\infty\left((1+s)^{H-\frac{1}{2}}-s^{H-\frac{1}{2}}\right)^2\,ds+\frac{1}{2H}\right)^{\frac{1}{2}}=\frac{(2H\sin(\pi H)\Gamma(2H))^{\frac{1}{2}}}{\Gamma(H+\frac{1}{2})},$$

see e.g. [8, Theorem 1.3.1].

There is another realization of fractional Brownian motion on the white noise space which is due to Bender:[1] Let $H\in(0,1)$, $I=[0,\infty)$ and

$$K_j(t,-)=M_-^H\mathbf{1}_{[0,t)}(-),\quad j=1,\ldots,d,$$

where

$$M_-^H f:=\begin{cases}\frac{(\frac{1}{2}-H)K_H}{\Gamma(H+\frac{1}{2})}\lim_{\varepsilon\searrow o}\int_\varepsilon^\infty\frac{f(x)-f(x+y)}{y^{\frac{3}{2}-H}}\,dy&,\text{ if }H\in(0,\frac{1}{2})\\[2mm]f&,\text{ if }H=\frac{1}{2}\\[2mm]\frac{K_H}{\Gamma(H-\frac{1}{2})}\int_x^\infty f(y)(y-x)^{H-\frac{3}{2}}\,dy&,\text{ if }H\in(\frac{1}{2},1).\end{cases}$$

Then, the stochastic process $\left(B_t^H\right)_{t \geq 0}$ with $B_t^H := \left\langle \cdot, M_-^H \mathbf{1}_{[0,t)} \right\rangle$ is a d-dimensional fractional Brownian motion with Hurst parameter H. This is due to the fact that for $H \in (0,1)$ and for all $t \in \mathbb{R}$

$$\left(M_-^{H-\frac{1}{2}} \mathbf{1}_{[0,t)}\right)(x) = \frac{1}{\Gamma(H+\frac{1}{2})} \left((t-x)_+^{H-\frac{1}{2}} - (-x)_+^{H-\frac{1}{2}}\right),$$

see e.g. [8, Lemma 1.1.3]. Moreover, we have the Bochner integral

$$\delta\left(\left\langle \cdot, M_-^H \mathbf{1}_{[0,t)} \right\rangle - c\right) := \left(\frac{1}{2\pi}\right)^d \int_{\mathbb{R}^d} \exp\left(i\lambda\left(\left\langle \cdot, M_-^H \mathbf{1}_{[0,t)} \right\rangle - c\right)\right) d\lambda$$

is a Hida distribution with S-transform given by

$$S\delta\left(\left\langle \cdot, M_-^H \mathbf{1}_{[0,t)} \right\rangle - c\right)\left(\vec{f}\right)$$

$$= \left(\frac{1}{\sqrt{2\pi t^{2H}}}\right)^d \exp\left(-\frac{1}{2t^{2H}} \sum_{j=1}^d \left(\int_0^t M_+^H f_j(x)\, dx - c_j\right)^2\right),$$

where

$$M_+^H f := \begin{cases} \frac{(\frac{1}{2}-H)K_H}{\Gamma(H+\frac{1}{2})} \lim_{\varepsilon \searrow o} \int_\varepsilon^\infty \frac{f(x)-f(x-y)}{y^{\frac{3}{2}-H}}\, dy & , \text{ if } H \in (0, \frac{1}{2}) \\ f & , \text{ if } H = \frac{1}{2} \\ \frac{K_H}{\Gamma(H-\frac{1}{2})} \int_{-\infty}^x f(y)(x-y)^{H-\frac{3}{2}}\, dy & , \text{ if } H \in (\frac{1}{2}, 1). \end{cases}$$

for all $\vec{f} \in \mathcal{S}_d(\mathbb{R})$. For $H \in (0, \frac{1}{2})$ $M_\pm^H$ is nothing else than the Marchaud fractional derivative operator and for $H \in (\frac{1}{2}, 1)$ $M_\pm^H$ is the Riemann-Weyl fractional integral operator. Note that for $f = \mathbf{1}_{[0,t)}$ or $f \in \mathcal{S}(\mathbb{R})$ it holds that $M_\pm^H f \in L^2(\mathbb{R})$. Note that by choosing $H = \frac{1}{2}$ we recover the classical Brownian motion.

(3) **Pure Volterra process**: In the preceding examples we only consider d-dimensional stochastic processes with d identical Volterra kernels in each coordinate. We can also consider d-dimensional pure Volterra process, i.e. we take different Volterra kernels which give different independent stochastic processes living in each coordinate of $\mathbb{R}^d$. As a simple example let $d = 2$, $K_1(t,s) = \mathbf{1}_{[0,t)}(s)$ and $K_2(t,s) = \mathbf{1}_{[0,t)}(s) - \frac{t}{T}\mathbf{1}_{[0,T)}(s)$. Then, the two-dimensional stochastic process

$$X = (X_t)_{t \in [0,T]} = \left(\left\langle \cdot, \mathbf{1}_{[0,t)} \right\rangle, \left\langle \cdot, \mathbf{1}_{[0,t)} - \frac{t}{T}\mathbf{1}_{[0,T)} \right\rangle\right)_{t \in [0,T]}$$

is a pure Volterra process with a Brownian motion in the first coordinate and a Brownian bridge (starting in 0 at time 0 and ending in 0 at time T) in the second coordinate.

4. Conclusion

We have presented some preliminary results on a white noise approach to Volterra processes. In particular, we discuss the Donsker delta function of Volterra processes as a white noise distribution. For future works we plan to consider the Volterra white noise, i.e. the generalized time derivative of a Volterra process, and some applications such as in the topics of local times, self-intersection local times and fractional path integral.

Acknowledgment

The author would like to thank Prof. Christopher C. Bernido and Prof. M. Victoria Carpio-Bernido for the invitation to the *7th Jagna International Workshop on Analysis of Fractional Stochastic Processes: Advances and Applications* and for their hospitality.

References

1. C. Bender, An Ito formula for generalized functionals of a fractional Brownian motion with arbitrary Hurst parameter, *Stoch. Proc. Appl.* **104**, 81–106, (2003).
2. F. Baudoin and D. Nualart, Equivalence of Volterra processes, *Stoch. Proc. Appl.* **107**, 327–350, (2003).
3. L. Decreusefond, Stochastic calculus with respect to Volterra processes, *Annales de l'Institut Henri Poincaré (B) Probability and Statistics* **41**, 123–149, (2005).
4. T. Hida, H-H. Kuo, J. Potthoff and L. Streit, *White Noise. An Infinite Dimensional Calculus*, (Kluwer Academic Publishers, Dordrecht, 1993).
5. H. Hult, Approximating some Volterra type stochastic integrals with applications to parameter estimation, *Stoch. Proc. Appl.* **105**, 1–32, (2003).
6. Y. Kondratiev, P. Leukert, J. Potthoff, L. Streit and W. Westerkamp, Generalized functionals in Gaussian spaces: The characterization theorem revisited, *J. Funct. Anal.* **141**, 301–318, (1996).
7. H-H. Kuo , *White Noise Distribution Theory*, (CRC Press, Boca Raton, 1996).
8. Y. Mishura, *Stochastic Calculus for Fractional Brownian Motion and Related Process*, (Springer, Heidelberg, 2008).
9. D. Nualart, A white noise approach to fractional Brownian motion, *Stochastic Analysis: Classical and Quantum. Perspectives of White Noise Theory*, 112–126, (2005).
10. N. Obata, *White Noise Calculus and Fock Space*, (Springer, Heidelberg, 1994).

7th Jagna International Workshop (2014)
International Journal of Modern Physics: Conference Series
Vol. 36 (2015) 1560006 (8 pages)
© The Authors
DOI: 10.1142/S201019451560006X

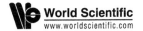
World Scientific
www.worldscientific.com

Stochastic path summation with memory

Christopher C. Bernido* and M. Victoria Carpio-Bernido

Research Center for Theoretical Physics,
Central Visayan Institute Foundation, Jagna, Bohol 6308, Philippines
*cbernido@mozcom.com

Published 2 January 2015

Some classes of stochastic processes with memory properties are investigated by evaluating the probability density function as a white noise path integral. The corresponding modified diffusion equation for different types of memory behavior is then discussed.

1. Introduction

Various natural and social phenomena are characterized by a degree of randomness and apparent memory of the past. Randomness, uncertainty, and stochasticity arise when too many unaccountable and undetermined factors affect the dynamical evolution of a system. Memory, on the other hand, manifests in emerging patterns and repetitions that could occur in an otherwise random development in time. Both stochasticity and memory, therefore, appear to be important ingredients in a mathematical model for phenomena at various scales. To incorporate these features, we take a variable x and express it in terms of the white noise random variable $\omega(t)$ and a memory function $f(T - t)$, where t is time which varies from 0 to T. We evaluate the probability density function as a sum-over-all histories[1-3] if x starts at x_0 and ends at x_T at time $t = T$. In particular, integration over all paths is done using the Gaussian white noise measure[4,5] $d\mu(\omega)$ where, $\omega = dB/dt$, with $B(t)$ a Wiener process. We then consider different types of memory behavior and mention some applications.

2. Parametrizing Stochasticity and Memory

To understand natural and social processes we normally track, observe, and record values of an important variable as it evolves in time. Designating this variable as x, its randomness and memory behavior may be parametrized as,[3,6]

$$x(T) = x_0 + \int_0^T f(T-t) \, h(t) \, \omega(t) \, dt \,, \tag{1}$$

where x_0 is the initial value, $f(T-t)$ is a memory function, and $h(t)$ is a time-dependent multiplying factor. Here, $\omega(t)$ is the Gaussian white noise variable defined such that ordinary Brownian motion is, $B(T) = \int_0^T \omega(t) \, dt$. As time t ranges from 0 to T in Eq. (1), the functions $f(T-t)$ and $h(t)$ modulate the random white noise variable $\omega(t)$ thereby affecting the value or history of $x(T)$. The explicit forms of $f(T-t)$ and $h(t)$ may be chosen depending on the system being modeled. For the special case where, $f(T-t) = h(t) = 1$, Eq. (1) reduces to the Markovian process,

$$x(T) = x_0 + B(T). \tag{2}$$

We now proceed to evaluate the transition probability for a system to go from x_0 to a specific endpoint, $x(T) = x_T$, at a later time $t = T$. As in the Feynman path integral,[1] randomness and uncertainty dictate that all possible paths starting from the intial point x_0 should be accommodated. However, only those paths which end at a given point x_T contribute in evaluating the transition probability (see, Fig. 1). This means that we consider only those paths which satisfy the delta function constraint,

$$\delta(x(T) - x_T) = \delta\left(x_0 + \int_0^T f(T-t) \, h(t) \, \omega(t) \, dt - x_T\right), \tag{3}$$

where we used Eq. (1) for $x(T)$.

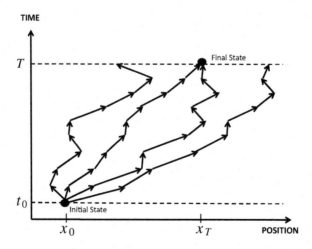

Fig. 1. At time $t = T$, paths may end at different points in space. The delta function constraint for paths on the left and right gives zero contribution. The two paths in the middle contribute to the probability density function.

The probability density function $P(x_T, T; x_0, 0)$ for paths satisfying the δ-function constraint can be obtained by evaluating the expectation value $E(\delta(x(T) - x_T))$ as,

$$
\begin{aligned}
P(x_T, T; x_0, 0) &= E(\delta(x(T) - x_T)) \\
&= \int \delta(x(T) - x_T) \, d\mu \\
&= \int \delta\left(x_0 + \int_0^T f(T-t) \, h(t) \, \omega(t) \, dt - x_T\right) d\mu,
\end{aligned}
$$

(4)

over the Gaussian white noise measure[5] $d\mu$.

Writing the delta function in terms of its Fourier representation we have,

$$
\begin{aligned}
P(x_T, T; x_0, 0) &= \frac{1}{2\pi} \int d\mu \int_{-\infty}^{+\infty} dk \\
&\quad \times \exp\left\{ik\left[\left(x_0 - x_T + \int_0^T f(T-t) \, h(t) \, \omega(t) \, dt\right)\right]\right\} \\
&= \frac{1}{2\pi} \int_{-\infty}^{+\infty} dk \exp\{ik[(x_0 - x_T)]\} \\
&\quad \times \int \exp\left\{ik \int_0^T f(T-t) \, h(t) \, \omega(t) \, dt\right\} d\mu \ .
\end{aligned}
$$

(5)

If we let, $\xi(t) = k \, f(T-t) \, h(t)$, the integration over $d\mu$ can be carried out, i.e.,[5]

$$
\int \exp\left\{i \int_0^T \omega(t) \xi(t) \, dt\right\} d\mu = \exp\left\{-\frac{1}{2} \int_0^T \xi^2(t) \, dt\right\} .
$$

(6)

Using this result in Eq. (5) we have,

$$
P(x_T, T; x_0, 0) = \int_{-\infty}^{+\infty} \frac{dk}{2\pi} \exp\left\{ik[(x_0 - x_T)] - \frac{k^2}{2} \int_0^T [f(T-t) \, h(t)]^2 \, dt\right\} .
$$

(7)

The integral over dk is a Gaussian integral which when evaluated yields the probability density function,

$$
\begin{aligned}
P(x_T, T; x_0, 0) &= \left(2\pi \int_0^T [f(T-t) \, h(t)]^2 \, dt\right)^{-\frac{1}{2}} \\
&\quad \times \exp\left(-\left[\int_0^T [f(T-t) \, h(t)]^2 \, dt\right]^{-1} \frac{(x_T - x_0)^2}{2}\right) .
\end{aligned}
$$

(8)

As a simple example, take the special case where $f(T-t)$ is just a constant, say, $f = \sqrt{2D}$ where D is a diffusion coefficient and $h(t) = 1$. Then, Eq. (8) reduces to the Gaussian distribution,

$$P(x_T, T; x_0, 0) = \frac{1}{\sqrt{4\pi DT}} \exp\left(\frac{-(x_T - x_0)^2}{4DT}\right), \tag{9}$$

which solves the diffusion equation for the Wiener process. Other examples are shown in the next section.

3. Memory Functions and Probability Densities

Using Eq. (8), we summarize in Table 1[6] some explicit examples of memory function $f(T-t)$ and $h(t)$ for which closed form solutions of the corresponding probability density function $P(x_T, T; x_0, 0)$ can be obtained. The equation numbers in the third column refer to Refs. 11 and 12.

4. Modified Diffusion Equation

We now look at the kinetic equation satisfied by the probability density function $P(x_T, T; x_0, 0)$ given by Eq. (8) with memory function $f(\tau - t)$. Using the notation, $x_T = x$, and $T = \tau$, the behavior of $P(x_T, T; x_0, 0)$ with respect to time can be seen by taking its time derivative,

$$\frac{\partial}{\partial \tau} P(x, \tau; x_0, 0) = \frac{\partial}{\partial \tau} \left\{ \frac{1}{\sqrt{2\pi \int_0^\tau [f(T-t)h(t)]^2\, dt}} \right.$$

$$\left. \times \exp\left[\frac{-(x-x_0)^2}{2\int_0^\tau [f(T-t)h(t)]^2\, dt} \right] \right\}, \tag{10}$$

which yields the expression,

$$\frac{\partial}{\partial \tau} P(x, \tau; x_0, 0) = \left[\frac{1}{2} \frac{\partial}{\partial \tau} \int_0^\tau [f(T-t)h(t)]^2\, dt \right]$$

$$\times \left\{ \frac{-P(x, \tau; x_0, 0)}{\int_0^\tau [f(T-t)h(t)]^2\, dt} \left[1 - \frac{(x-x_0)^2}{\int_0^\tau [f(T-t)h(t)]^2\, dt} \right] \right\}. \tag{11}$$

On the other hand, an evaluation of, $(\partial^2/\partial x^2)P(x, \tau; x_0, 0)$, using Eq. (8) shows that it is equal to the factor in curly brackets in Eq. (11), in particular,

$$\frac{\partial^2}{\partial x^2} P(x, \tau; x_0, 0) = \frac{-P(x, \tau; x_0, 0)}{\int_0^\tau [f(T-t)h(t)]^2\, dt} \left[1 - \frac{(x-x_0)^2}{\int_0^\tau [f(T-t)h(t)]^2\, dt} \right]. \tag{12}$$

Table 1. Memory function with corresponding Probability Density Function. Equation numbers are those in Refs. 11 and 12.

Memory Function $f(T-t)$	$h(t)$	Probability Density Function $P(x_T, T; x_0, 0)$
[1] $f = \frac{(T-t)^{H-1/2}}{\Gamma(H+1/2)}$	$h = 1$	$\sqrt{\dfrac{H\,\Gamma^2\left(H+\frac{1}{2}\right)}{\pi T^{2H}}}$ $\times \exp\left(-\dfrac{H\,\Gamma^2\left(H+\frac{1}{2}\right)(x_0-x_T)^2}{T^{2H}}\right)$
[2] $f = \sin^{\frac{1}{2}}(T-t)$	$h = \sqrt{J_0(t)}$	$[2\pi T J_1(T)]^{-\frac{1}{2}} \exp\left(-\dfrac{(x_T-x_0)^2}{2T J_1(T)}\right)$ Eq. (6.674.7) of Ref.11
[3] $f = \cos^{\frac{1}{2}}(T-t)$	$h = \sqrt{J_0(t)}$	$[2\pi T J_0(T)]^{-\frac{1}{2}} \exp\left(-\dfrac{(x_T-x_0)^2}{2T J_0(T)}\right)$ Eq. (6.674.8) of Ref. 11
[4] $f = (T-t)^{\frac{\mu-1}{2}}$ $[\mathrm{Re}\,\mu > 0,\ T > 0]$	$h = \dfrac{e^{-\beta/2t}}{t^{(\mu+1)/2}}$	$\dfrac{\beta^{\mu/2}e^{\beta/2T}}{\sqrt{2\pi}\Gamma(\mu)T^{\mu-1}} \exp\left(-\dfrac{\beta^\mu e^{\beta/T}(x_T-x_0)^2}{2\,\Gamma(\mu)\,T^{\mu-1}}\right)$ Eq. (3.471.3) of Ref. 11
[5] $f = (T-t)^{\frac{\mu-1}{2}}$ $[\mathrm{Re}\,\mu > 0,\ T > 0]$	$h = \dfrac{e^{-\beta/2t}}{t^{(1-\nu)/2}}$ $[\mathrm{Re}\,\beta > 0]$	$\dfrac{T^{\frac{1-2\mu-\nu}{4}}e^{\frac{\beta}{4T}}}{\sqrt{2\pi\beta^{\frac{\nu-1}{2}}\Gamma(\mu)W_{\frac{1-2\mu-\nu}{2},\frac{\nu}{2}}\left(\frac{\beta}{T}\right)}}$ $\times \exp\left(\dfrac{-\beta^{\frac{1-\nu}{2}}T^{\frac{1-2\mu-\nu}{2}}e^{\frac{\beta}{2T}}(x_T-x_0)^2}{2\Gamma(\mu)W_{\frac{1-2\mu-\nu}{2},\frac{\nu}{2}}\left(\frac{\beta}{T}\right)}\right)$ Eq. (3.471.2) of Ref. 11
[6] $f = (T-t)^{\frac{\mu-1}{2}}$ $[\mathrm{Re}\,\mu > 0,\ T > 0]$	$h = \dfrac{e^{-\beta/2t}}{t^\mu}$ $[\mathrm{Re}\,\beta > 0]$	$\dfrac{1}{\sqrt{2\sqrt{\frac{\pi}{T}}\beta^{\frac{1}{2}-\mu}e^{-\frac{\beta}{2T}}\Gamma(\mu)K_{\mu-\frac{1}{2}}\left(\frac{\beta}{2T}\right)}}$ $\times \exp\left(\dfrac{-\sqrt{\pi T}(x_T-x_0)^2}{2\beta^{\frac{1}{2}-\mu}e^{-\frac{\beta}{2T}}\Gamma(\mu)K_{\mu-\frac{1}{2}}\left(\frac{\beta}{2T}\right)}\right)$ Eq. (3.471.4) of Ref. 11
[7] $f = (T-t)^{\frac{\mu-1}{2}}$ $[\mathrm{Re}\,\mu > 0]$	$h = \dfrac{e^{\beta t/2}}{t^{(1-\nu)/2}}$ $[\mathrm{Re}\,\nu > 0]$	$\dfrac{1}{\sqrt{2\pi B(\mu,\nu)T^{T+\nu-1}\,_1F_1(\nu;\mu+\nu;\beta T)}}$ $\times \exp\left(\dfrac{-(x_T-x_0)^2}{2B(\mu,\nu)T^{T+\nu-1}\,_1F_1(\nu;\mu+\nu;\beta T)}\right)$ Eq. (3.383.1) of Ref. 11
[8] $f = (T-t)^{\frac{\mu-1}{2}}$ $[\mathrm{Re}\,\mu > 0]$	$h = \dfrac{e^{\beta t/2}}{t^{(1-\mu)/2}}$	$\dfrac{1}{\sqrt{2\pi^{\frac{3}{2}}\left(\frac{T}{\beta}\right)^{T-\frac{1}{2}}e^{\left(\frac{\beta T}{2}\right)}\Gamma(\mu)I_{\mu-\frac{1}{2}}\left(\frac{\beta T}{2}\right)}}$ $\times \exp\left(\dfrac{-\left(\frac{T}{\beta}\right)^{\frac{1}{2}-T}(x_T-x_0)^2}{2\sqrt{\pi}e^{\left(\frac{\beta T}{2}\right)}\Gamma(\mu)I_{\mu-\frac{1}{2}}\left(\frac{\beta T}{2}\right)}\right)$ Eq. (3.383.2) of Ref. 11
[9] $f = (T-t)^{\frac{\mu-1}{2}}$ $[\mathrm{Re}\,\mu > 0]$	$h = \dfrac{\sin^{\frac{1}{2}}(at)}{t^{\frac{1-\mu}{2}}}$	$\sqrt{\dfrac{\pi^{-3/2}T^{\frac{1}{2}-\mu}a^{\mu-\frac{1}{2}}}{2\sin\left(\frac{aT}{2}\right)\Gamma(\mu)J_{\mu-\frac{1}{2}}\left(\frac{aT}{2}\right)}}$ $\times \exp\left(-\dfrac{\pi^{-\frac{1}{2}}T^{\frac{1}{2}-\mu}a^{\mu-\frac{1}{2}}(x_0-x_T)^2}{2\sin\left(\frac{aT}{2}\right)\Gamma(\mu)J_{\mu-\frac{1}{2}}\left(\frac{aT}{2}\right)}\right)$ Eq. (3.768.7) of Ref. 11

Table 1. (*Continued*)

Memory Function $f(T-t)$	$h(t)$	Probability Density Function $P(x_T, T; x_0, 0)$
[10] $f = (T-t)^{\frac{\mu-1}{2}}$ [Re $\mu > 0$]	$h = \dfrac{\cos^{\frac12}(at)}{t^{\frac{1-\mu}{2}}}$	$\sqrt{\dfrac{\pi^{-3/2}T^{\frac12-\mu}a^{\mu-\frac12}}{2\cos(\frac{aT}{2})\Gamma(\mu)J_{\mu-\frac12}(\frac{aT}{2})}}$ $\times \exp\left(-\dfrac{\pi^{-\frac12}T^{\frac12-\mu}a^{\mu-\frac12}(x_0-x_T)^2}{2\cos(\frac{aT}{2})\Gamma(\mu)J_{\mu-\frac12}(\frac{aT}{2})}\right)$ Eq. (3.768.9) of Ref. 11
[11] $f = (T-t)^{\frac{\mu-1}{2}}$ [Re$\mu > 0$]	$h = \dfrac{(t^2+\beta^2)^{\frac{\nu}{2}}}{t^{\frac{1-\lambda}{2}}}$ [$\lambda > 0$]	$\sqrt{\dfrac{\beta^{-2\nu}T^{1-\lambda-\mu}}{2\pi B(\lambda,\mu)\,_3F_2\left(-\nu,\frac{\lambda}{2},\frac{\lambda+1}{2};\frac{\lambda+\mu}{2},\frac{\lambda+\mu+1}{2};\frac{-T^2}{\beta^2}\right)}}$ $\times \exp\left(\dfrac{-[B(\lambda,\mu)]^{-1}\beta^{-2\nu}T^{1-\lambda-\mu}(x_0-x_T)^2}{2\,_3F_2\left(-\nu,\frac{\lambda}{2},\frac{\lambda+1}{2};\frac{\lambda+\mu}{2},\frac{\lambda+\mu+1}{2};\frac{-T^2}{\beta^2}\right)}\right)$ $\left[\text{Re}\left(\frac{T}{\beta}\right) > 0\right]$; Eq. (3.254.1) of Ref. 11
[12] $f = (T-t)^{-\frac{\nu}{2}}$ [$|\text{Re }\nu| < 1$]	$h = \sqrt{\dfrac{(t-a)^\nu}{(t-c)}}$ [$c < T$]	$\dfrac{1}{\pi\sqrt{2\csc(\nu\pi)\left[1-\cos(\nu\pi)\left(\frac{c}{T-c}\right)^\nu\right]}}$ $\times \exp\left(\dfrac{-\csc^{-1}(\nu\pi)(x_T-x_0)^2}{2\pi\left[1-\cos(\nu\pi)\left(\frac{c}{T-c}\right)^\nu\right]}\right)$ Eq. (3.228.1) of Ref. 11
[13] $f = (T-t)^{-\nu/2}$ [$0.5 < \text{Re }\nu < 1$]	$h = \sqrt{\dfrac{(t-a)^{\nu-1}}{(t-c)}}$ [$c < T$]	$\sqrt{\dfrac{(T-c)^\nu}{-2\pi^2(c)^{\nu-1}\cot(\nu\pi)}}$ $\times \exp\left(\dfrac{(T-c)^\nu(x_T-x_0)^2}{2\pi(c)^{\nu-1}\cot(\nu\pi)}\right)$ Eq. (3.228.2) of Ref. 11
[14] $f = (T-t)^{\nu/2}$ [Re $\nu > -1$, $T > 0$]	$h = e^{-\mu t/2}$	$\dfrac{1}{\sqrt{2\pi(-\mu)^{-\nu-1}e^{-T\mu}\,\gamma(\nu+1,-T\mu)}}$ $\times \exp\left(\dfrac{-e^{T\mu}(x_T-x_0)^2}{2(-\mu)^{-\nu-1}\gamma(\nu+1,-T\mu)}\right)$ Eq. (3.382.1) of Ref. 11
[15] $f = \sqrt{J_{1-\nu}(T-t)}$ [$-1 < \text{Re}\nu < 2$]	$h = \sqrt{J_\nu(t)}$	$\dfrac{1}{\sqrt{2\pi(J_0(T)-\cos T)}}$ $\times \exp\left(\dfrac{-(x_T-x_0)^2}{2(J_0(T)-\cos T)}\right)$ Eq. (11.3.38) of Ref. 12
[16] $f = \sqrt{J_\nu(T-t)}$ [Re$\nu > -1$]	$h = \sqrt{t^{-1}J_\mu(t)}$ [Re$\mu > 0$]	$\sqrt{\dfrac{\mu}{2\pi J_{\mu+\nu}(T)}}$ $\times \exp\left(\dfrac{-\mu(x_T-x_0)^2}{2J_{\mu+\nu}(T)}\right)$ Eq. (11.3.40) of Ref. 12

Using Eq. (12) on the right-hand-side of Eq. (11) yields a modified diffusion equation (13) satisfied by $P(x,\tau;x_0,0)$, i.e.,

$$\frac{\partial}{\partial\tau}P(x,\tau;x_0,0) = \left[\frac{1}{2}\frac{\partial}{\partial\tau}\int_0^\tau [f(T-t)\,h(t)]^2\,dt\right]\frac{\partial^2}{\partial x^2}P(x,\tau;x_0,0), \qquad (13)$$

where, instead of a constant diffusion coefficient, a time-dependent diffusive behavior is allowed.[13] We now look at specific examples where the corresponding solution $P(x,\tau;x_0,0)$ has been applied to actual physical systems.[10,14]

(a) Ordinary Brownian Motion:

Consider the special case where $f(T-t)$ is just a constant given by $f = \sqrt{2D}$ and $h(t) = 1$. Eq. (13) yields,

$$\frac{\partial}{\partial \tau} P(x, \tau; x_0, 0) = D \frac{\partial^2}{\partial x^2} P(x, \tau; x_0, 0) \tag{14}$$

which is the usual diffusion equation for the Wiener process where D is a diffusion coefficient.

(b) Fractional Brownian Motion:

For a memory function $f(T-t)$ and $h(t) = 1$ given by number (1) in Table 1 of the previous section, we have,

$$\frac{\partial}{\partial \tau} \int_0^\tau [f(T-t) h(t)]^2 \, dt = \frac{\partial}{\partial \tau} \left(\frac{\tau^{2H}}{2H \, \Gamma \left(H + \frac{1}{2} \right)^2} \right)$$

$$= \frac{\tau^{2H-1}}{\Gamma \left(H + \frac{1}{2} \right)^2}. \tag{15}$$

Using this in Eq. (13) yields,

$$\frac{\partial}{\partial \tau} P(x, \tau; x_0, 0) = \frac{\tau^{2H-1}}{2\Gamma \left(H + \frac{1}{2} \right)^2} \frac{\partial^2}{\partial x^2} P(x, \tau; x_0, 0), \tag{16}$$

which is the diffusion equation for fractional Brownian motion in Riemann-Liouville representation.[2]

(c) Exponentially-modified Brownian Motion:

For the memory function $f(\tau - t)$ and $h(t)$ described by entry [4] in Table 1 we have,

$$\frac{\partial}{\partial \tau} \int_0^\tau [f(\tau - t) h(t)]^2 \, dt = \frac{\partial}{\partial \tau} \int_0^\tau (\tau - t)^{\mu-1} \left(\frac{e^{-\beta/t}}{t^{\mu+1}} \right) dt$$

$$= \frac{\partial}{\partial \tau} \left(\frac{\Gamma(\mu) \tau^{\mu-1} e^{-\beta/\tau}}{\beta^\mu} \right)$$

$$= \frac{\Gamma(\mu) e^{-\beta/\tau}}{\beta^\mu} \left[(\mu - 1) \tau^{\mu-2} + \beta \tau^{\mu-3} \right]. \tag{17}$$

This gives rise to a modified diffusion equation of the form,

$$\frac{\partial}{\partial \tau} P(x, \tau; x_0, 0) = \left(\frac{\Gamma(\mu) e^{-\beta/\tau}}{2\beta^\mu} \left[(\mu - 1) \tau^{\mu-2} + \beta \tau^{\mu-3} \right] \right) \frac{\partial^2}{\partial x^2} P(x, \tau; x_0, 0). \tag{18}$$

5. Conclusion

The sum-over-all-paths approach to describe stochastic processes possessing various types of memory behavior allows a wider range of real-world applications. One advantage of the path integral is its ability to handle systems with boundaries and spaces with topological constraints[6, 15, 16] often encountered in actual experiments. The wide array of possible memory functions is also an advantage in dealing with the diversity of natural and social phenomena. Applications could range from complex systems to microrheology and neurophysics, going beyond the mathematically well-studied fractional Brownian motion.[6–10, 14]

Acknowledgments

The authors gratefully acknowledge the Alexander von Humboldt Foundation and Prof. L. Streit for research visits at Universität Bielefeld.

References

1. R. P. Feynman and A. R. Hibbs, *Quantum Mechanics and Path Integrals* (McGraw-Hill, New York, 1965).
2. I. Calvo and R. Sánchez, The path integral formulation of fractional Brownian motion for the general Hurst exponent, *J. Phys. A: Math. Theor.* **41** (2008) 282002.
3. C. C. Bernido and M. V. Carpio-Bernido, White noise analysis: some applications in complex systems, biophysics and quantum mechanics, *Int. Jour. Mod. Phys. B* **26** (2012) 1230014.
4. L. Streit and T. Hida, Generalized Brownian functionals and the Feynman integral, *Stoch. Proc. Appl.* **16** (1983) 55–69.
5. T. Hida, H. H. Kuo, J. Potthoff, L. Streit, *White Noise. An Infinite Dimensional Calculus* (Kluwer, Dordrecht, 1993).
6. C. C. Bernido and M. V. Carpio-Bernido, *Methods and Applications of White Noise Analysis in Interdisciplinary Sciences* (World Scientific, Singapore, 2014).
7. S. C. Lim and S. V. Muniandy, Self-similar Gaussian processes for modeling anomalous diffusion, *Phys. Rev. E* **66** (2002) 021114.
8. Y. Mishura, *Stochastic Calculus for Fractional Brownian Motion and Related Processes*, (Springer-Verlag, Berlin, 2008).
9. J. Klafter, S. C. Lim, R. Metzler, eds., *Fractional Dynamics* (World Scientific, Singapore, 2012).
10. F. Biagini, Y. Hu, B. Øksendal and T. Zhang, *Stochastic Calculus for Fractional Brownian Motion and Applications* (Springer-Verlag, London, 2008).
11. I. S. Gradshteyn and I. M. Ryzhik, *Table of Integrals, Series and Products*, 5th edition (Academic Press, San Diego, 1994).
12. M. Abramowitz and I. A. Stegun: *Handbook of Mathematical Functions with Formulas, Graphs, and Mathematical Tables* (National Bureau of Standards, Washington D. C., 1972) p. 485.
13. K. G. Wang and C. W. Lung, Long-time correlation effects and fractal Brownian motion, *Phys. Lett. A* **151** (1990) 119-121.
14. C. C. Bernido, M. V. Carpio-Bernido, and M. G. O. Escobido, Modified diffusion with memory for cyclone track fluctuations, *Phys. Lett. A* **378** (2014) 2016–2019; **379** (2015) 230–231.
15. L. S. Schulman, *Techniques and Applications of Path Integration* (Wiley, New York, 1981).
16. C. Grosche and F. Steiner, *Handbook of Feynman Path Integrals* (Springer, Berlin, 1998).

7th Jagna International Workshop (2014)
International Journal of Modern Physics: Conference Series
Vol. 36 (2015) 1560007 (16 pages)
© The Author
DOI: 10.1142/S2010194515600071

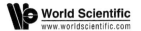
World Scientific
www.worldscientific.com

Weak ergodicity breaking and ageing in anomalous diffusion

Ralf Metzler

*Institute for Physics & Astronomy, University of Potsdam,
D-14476 Potsdam-Golm, Germany & Department of Physics,
Tampere University of Technology, FI-33101 Tampere, Finland*

Published 2 January 2015

Modern single particle tracking techniques and many large scale simulations produce time series $\mathbf{r}(t)$ of the position of a tracer particle. Standardly these are evaluated in terms of the time averaged mean squared displacement. For ergodic processes such as Brownian motion, one can interpret the results of such an analysis in terms of the known theories for the corresponding ensemble averaged mean squared displacement, if only the measurement time is sufficiently long. In anomalous diffusion processes, that are widely observed over many orders of magnitude, the equivalence between (long) time and ensemble averages may be broken (weak ergodicity breaking). In such cases the time averages may no longer be interpreted in terms of ensemble theories. Here we collect some recent results on weakly non-ergodic systems with respect to the time averaged mean squared displacement and the inherent irreproducibility of individual measurements. We also address the phenomenon of ageing, the dependence of physical observables on the time span between initial preparation of the system and the start of the measurement.

Keywords: Anomalous diffusion; ensemble average; time average; ageing; non-stationarity.

1. Introduction

Following the three groundbreaking papers on the theory of Brownian motion[1] by Albert Einstein,[2] Marian Smoluchowski,[3] and Paul Langevin,[4] in 1908 Jean Perrin reported the first systematic single particle tracking results in his seminal paper on diffusion. Perrin used microscopic diffusion measurements of small putty particles to determine Avogadro's number via the Einstein-Stokes-Smoluchowski relation.[5] Due to the relatively short trajectories, Perrin used the ensemble information of many measured, not completely identical particles in his analysis.[5] Only six years after Perrin's first publication and exactly hundred years ago, in 1914 Ivar Nordlund conceived an experimental setup, that allowed him to record long time traces of

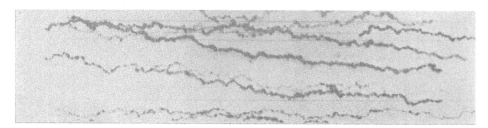

Fig. 1. Sample trajectories of sedimenting mercury droplets measured by Ivar Nordlund in 1914 with his moving film technique, time increases to the right.[6] The jiggly motion of the droplets superimposed onto the deterministic sedimentation shows the Brownian motion of the droplets.

small mercury droplets on a moving film. From the records he then evaluated single particle trajectories in terms of *time averages* of the mean squared displacement.[6] Figure 1 shows typical trajectories measured by Nordlund.[6] His method was continuously refined in the following two decades, culminating in the measurements of Eugen Kappler,[7] whose result for Avogadro's number is within 1% of the current best known value.

Single particle tracking has become a routine tool in living biological cells as well as complex fluids *in vitro*.[8] Common tracer particles include fluorescently labelled molecules such as messenger RNA in the cytoplasm of cells or protein channels in their membranes. Without labels, submicron tracers such as endogenous granules or internalised particles such as viruses or plastic spheres can be directly monitored in microscopes.

Consider first a passive tracer particle in a simple liquid such as water. Single particle tracking of this tracer will reproduce the laws of Brownian motion. The ensemble averaged mean squared displacement (MSD)

$$\langle \mathbf{r}^2(t) \rangle = \int \mathbf{r}^2 P(\mathbf{r}, t) d\mathbf{r} \tag{1}$$

obtained as average of $\mathbf{r}^2$ over the probability density function $P(\mathbf{r}, t)$ will yield the linear scaling $\langle \mathbf{r}^2(t) \rangle \simeq K_1 t$ with time t, where K_1 is the diffusion constant. The proportionality factor depends on the spatial dimension. Single particle tracking experiments produce the time series $\mathbf{r}(t)$ of the particle position. Typically, few but long trajectories $\mathbf{r}(t)$ are measured and analysed in terms of the time averaged MSD

$$\overline{\delta^2(\Delta)} = \frac{1}{T - \Delta} \int_0^{T-\Delta} \left[\mathbf{r}(t + \Delta) - \mathbf{r}(t) \right]^2 dt. \tag{2}$$

This moving average sums the particle displacements within the lag time Δ over the time series $\mathbf{r}(t)$ of length (measurement time) T. For normal Brownian motion, the long time limit yields[9]

$$\overline{\delta^2(\Delta)} \simeq K_1 \Delta, \tag{3}$$

and we find the equivalence $\langle \mathbf{r}^2(\Delta) \rangle = \overline{\delta^2(\Delta)}$ of ensemble and time averaged MSDs. This is a restatement of Boltzmann's ergodic hypothesis: long time and ensemble averages of physical observables are equivalent. In the following we will also consider the average over individual trajectories,

$$\left\langle \overline{\delta^2(\Delta)} \right\rangle = \frac{1}{N} \sum_{i=1}^{N} \overline{\delta_i^2(\Delta)} = \frac{1}{T-\Delta} \int_0^{T-\Delta} \left\langle \left[\mathbf{r}(t+\Delta) - \mathbf{r}(t) \right]^2 \right\rangle dt. \tag{4}$$

In many systems deviations from Brownian motion are observed. This anomalous diffusion is typically of the power-law form[10]

$$\langle \mathbf{r}^2(t) \rangle \simeq K_\alpha t^\alpha \tag{5}$$

with the anomalous diffusion exponent α and the generalised diffusion coefficient K_α of physical dimension $[K_\alpha] = \mathrm{cm}^2/\mathrm{sec}^\alpha$. We distinguish subdiffusion ($0 < \alpha < 1$) and superdiffusion ($\alpha > 1$). Anomalous diffusion is often measured in crowded media, in particular, in living biological cells.[11–14]

Anomalous diffusion loses the universality of Brownian motion, and the MSD (5) is no longer sufficient to uniquely identify a stochastic process. Many different stochastic processes give rise to anomalous diffusion, and they exhibit many different features. The question we address here is the violation of ergodicity: we analyse which processes give rise to the disparity $\langle \mathbf{r}^2(\Delta) \rangle \neq \overline{\delta^2(\Delta)}$ and related properties. As we will see, several commonly used anomalous stochastic processes violate ergodicity and effect the irreproducibility of single particle tracking measurements.

2. Fractional Brownian and Langevin Equation Motion

The well known Langevin equation in the overdamped limit[a]

$$\frac{dx(t)}{dt} = \sqrt{2K_1} \times \xi(t) \tag{6}$$

is driven by white Gaussian noise of zero mean and correlator $\langle \xi(t)\xi(t') \rangle \sim \delta(t - t')$.[4,15] In contrast to the δ-correlation fractional Gaussian noise (fGn) has the power-law correlation

$$\langle \xi(t)\xi(t') \rangle \sim \alpha K_\alpha(\alpha - 1)|t - t'|^{\alpha-2}, \tag{7}$$

with exponent $0 < \alpha < 2$. FGn is known to characterise the tracer motion in viscoelastic environments.[16–21] Such correlated noise also governs the motion of individual lipids in lipid membranes,[22–24] and fGn occurs for the motion of a tracer particle in a single file of colloidal particles with excluded volume interactions.[25] In the case $0 < \alpha < 1$ the noise-noise correlator has a negative sign, a situation often termed antipersistent noise. In the case $1 < \alpha < 2$ we speak of persistence.

---

[a]For simplicity, we will use the one-dimensional notation for the remainder of this chapter.

2.1. *Fractional Brownian motion (FBM)*

Fractional Brownian motion simply substitutes the white Gaussian noise in the Langevin equation (6) with fGn (7).[26, 27] From a physical point of view, fGn is to be considered an external noise. The resulting ensemble average for the MSD is given by Eq. (5). FBM is ergodic in the sense that the time averaged MSD for unconfined motion becomes[28]

$$\overline{\delta^2(\Delta)} \sim 2K_\alpha \Delta^\alpha \tag{8}$$

in the limit of long T. We emphasise that the equality $\overline{\delta^2(\Delta)} = \langle x^2(\Delta) \rangle$ indeed holds for a single trajectory in the long measurement time T limit,[16] as expected for an ergodic process. The approach to ergodicity occurs as a power-law, similar to regular Brownian motion.[28]

In addition to the ergodic behaviour, individual trajectories of FBM are reproducible. More precisely, the amplitude variation of the time averaged MSD $\overline{\delta^2(\Delta)}$ from different realisations of length T around the mean $\langle \overline{\delta^2(\Delta)} \rangle$ is Gaussian. At a fixed lag time Δ, the width of this distribution decreases with increasing measurement time T,[29] and sufficiently long individual trajectories are therefore in that sense reproducible.

2.2. *Fractional Langevin equation motion*

When we require that the fGn is internal and should fulfil the Kubo generalised fluctuation-dissipation theorem, the resulting particle motion in the overdamped limit is described by the fractional Langevin equation (FLE)[30]

$$\gamma \int_0^t (t - t')^{\alpha-2} \frac{dx(t')}{dt'} dt' = \sqrt{\frac{\gamma k_B \mathscr{T}}{\alpha(\alpha - 1)K_\alpha}} \times \xi(t), \tag{9}$$

for $1 < \alpha < 2$. Here $k_B \mathscr{T}$ represents the thermal energy. In this formulation the long-range correlations of the noise are matched by the memory integral over the friction kernel. In terms of the fractional Caputo derivative[31]

$$\frac{d^{2-\alpha}x(t)}{dt^{2-\alpha}} = \frac{1}{\Gamma(\alpha - 1)} \int_0^t (t - t')^{\alpha-2} \frac{dx(t')}{dt'} dt'. \tag{10}$$

Eq. (9) can be rewritten in the compact form

$$\frac{d^{2-\alpha}x(t)}{dt^{2-\alpha}} = \frac{1}{\Gamma(\alpha - 1)} \sqrt{\frac{k_B \mathscr{T}}{\gamma\alpha(\alpha - 1)K_\alpha}} \times \xi(t), \tag{11}$$

hence the name fractional Langevin equation.[32] FLE motion is ergodic,

$$\overline{\delta^2(\Delta, T)} \sim \langle x^2(\Delta) \rangle \simeq 2K_{2-\alpha} \Delta^{2-\alpha}. \tag{12}$$

Due to the restriction $1 < \alpha < 2$, FLE motion is therefore subdiffusive. As for FBM, the approach to ergodicity is algebraic.[28] We note that FLE motion was also used recently in models of active transport in living cells.[33]

2.3. *Transient non-ergodicity of FBM & FLE motion*

The MSD for both FBM and FLE motion crosses over to a plateau in confinement, for instance, in case of diffusion in an harmonic potential $V(x) = kx^2/2$.[34] In the case of FBM, no temperature is defined, and the value of the plateau is a function of the anomalous diffusion exponent α, $\langle x^2 \rangle_{\mathrm{st}} = K_\alpha \Gamma(1 + \alpha)/k^\alpha$.[35] The associated time averaged MSD becomes $\langle \overline{\delta^2}_{\mathrm{stat}} \rangle = 2\langle x^2 \rangle_{\mathrm{st}}$. Here the factor two between the MSD and the time averaged MSD is due to the definition (2), which involves twice the stationary value $\langle x^2 \rangle_{\mathrm{st}}$.[36] In contrast to FBM, FLE motion fulfils the fluctuation-dissipation relation, and the MSD relaxes to the unique plateau value $\langle x^2 \rangle_{\mathrm{th}} = k_B \mathscr{T}/k$, while the time average converges to $\langle \overline{\delta^2}_{\mathrm{th}} \rangle = 2\langle x^2 \rangle_{\mathrm{th}}$.[36]

While for the free FBM and FLE motion ergodic behaviour is found the crossover to the stationary plateau turns out to be transiently non-ergodic. For both FBM and FLE motion the relaxation of the ensemble averaged MSD is exponential. However, for the time averaged MSD the approach is algebraic. For FBM we find[36]

$$\overline{\delta^2(\Delta)} \sim 2\langle x^2 \rangle_{\mathrm{st}} - \frac{K_\alpha \Gamma(\alpha + 1)}{k^2} e^{-k\Delta} - \frac{2\alpha(\alpha - 1)K_\alpha}{k^2 \Delta^{2-\alpha}}, \tag{13}$$

and for FLE motion[36]

$$\overline{\delta^2(\Delta)} \sim 2\langle x^2 \rangle_{\mathrm{th}} \left(1 - \frac{\gamma}{k\Delta^{2-\alpha}}\right). \tag{14}$$

This transient weak ergodicity breaking may lead to the false assumption that in the analysis of data the process has not yet relaxed, while the corresponding MSD $\langle x^2(t) \rangle$ already reached the plateau. This algebraic return to the ergodic behaviour represented by the plateau reminds of the algebraic approach to ergodicity of the free motion mentioned above. For single particle tracking experiments of submicron tracer beads in a worm-like micellar solution, this behaviour is indeed shown in Fig. 2. In this example the confinement is exerted by the optical tweezers used to track the particle.[19]

2.4. *Transient ageing of FBM & FLE motion*

What happens when the system is initially prepared at time $t = 0$ and we start the measurement at some later time $t_a > 0$, the ageing time? We then define the time averaged MSD as[37,38]

$$\overline{\delta^2(\Delta)} = \frac{1}{T - \Delta} \int_{t_a}^{t_a + T - \Delta} \left[x(t + \Delta) - x(t)\right]^2 dt. \tag{15}$$

A Brownian system naturally shows no dependence on t_a. Even though the process is asymptotically ergodic, however, we observe a transient dependence on t_a for processes driven by fGn. In general, for these processes it is found that the time average MSD always contains the two additive terms,[37]

$$\left\langle \overline{\delta^2(\Delta)} \right\rangle = f_{\mathrm{st}}(\Delta) + f_{\mathrm{age}}(\Delta; t_a, T). \tag{16}$$

The stationary term depends only on Δ, while the second, ageing term explicitly depends on T and t_a.

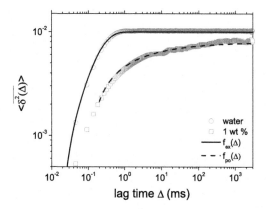

Fig. 2.   The time averaged MSD of submicron tracer beads in water (circles) and a viscoelastic solution with 1% worm-like micelles (squares).[19] The measurement is based on optical tweezers tracking, so that the initial free motion of the tracer bead eventually becomes confined by the tweezers potential. The time averaged MSD in water relaxes exponentially (full line), while in the worm-like micellar solution we observe the algebraic relaxation of Eq. (14), shown by the dashed line.

Free FLE motion has a stationary term featuring subdiffusion, $f_{\mathrm{st}} \simeq \Delta^{2-\alpha}$, and the ageing term decays as $f_{\mathrm{age}} \simeq 1/T$ as long as the initial velocity distribution is not thermal. In the limit $t_a \gg T$, we find the ageing time dependence[37]

$$f_{\mathrm{age}} \simeq t_a^{-2\alpha}. \qquad (17)$$

Under confinement FLE motion the term f_{st} has a power-law approach to the thermal plateau value, while again $f_{\mathrm{age}} \simeq 1/T$. Interestingly, a different t_a-scaling is followed by the ageing term,[37]

$$f_{\mathrm{age}} \simeq t_a^{2\alpha-6}. \qquad (18)$$

Confined FBM has $f_{\mathrm{age}} \simeq 1/T$, however, the ageing term shows the exponential decay[37]

$$f_{\mathrm{age}} \sim x_0^2 \exp(-2kt_a). \qquad (19)$$

3. Subdiffusive Continuous Time Random Walks

As discussed in the previous section, FBM and FLE motion reach the ergodic behaviour algebraically, similar to Brownian motion. For sufficiently long measurements, individual trajectories become fully reproducible, and ergodicity is achieved in every single trajectory. Here we introduce a process, for which ergodicity is broken asymptotically, and even for long measurement times T individual trajectories never become reproducible. This process is the well-known Scher-Montroll-Weiss continuous time random walk (CTRW):[39–41] after each jump a random walker is trapped (immobilised) for some waiting time t before it is allowed to jump again. The waiting times t are independent random variables, that is, CTRWs are renewal processes. Waiting times are distributed identically with the waiting time probability density function $\psi(t)$. The form proposed originally by Scher and Montroll is the power-law[40]

$$\psi(t) \simeq \frac{\tau^\alpha}{t^{1+\alpha}}, \quad 0 < \alpha < 1. \tag{20}$$

With this distribution of waiting times, the process leads to the subdiffusive MSD (5).[40,41] Due to the range of α, no characteristic waiting time $\langle t \rangle = \int_0^\infty t\psi(t)dt \to \infty$ exists. This scale-free nature of the CTRW process no longer possesses a time scale that allows one to distinguish a single or few jumps from many jumps. Typically, in a given trajectory longer and longer individual waiting events occur which can become of the order of the measurement time T, no matter how long we run the measurement.

CTRW-type stochastic motion was observed in a wide range of systems, spanning the motion of charge carriers in amorphous semiconductors,[40] the dispersion of tracer chemicals in subsurface aquifers,[42] as well as the motion of tracer beads in cross-linked semiflexible actin gels[43] and of functionalised colloidal particles facing complementarily functionalised surfaces.[44] In living cells, the motion of lipid and insulin granules in the cell cytoplasm[17,18] as well as of protein channels in the plasma membrane[45] follow the law (20).

The lack of a characteristic waiting time scale effects weak ergodicity breaking,[46,47] and the time averaged MSD becomes[48,49]

$$\left\langle \overline{\delta^2(\Delta)} \right\rangle \sim 2 \frac{K_\alpha}{\Gamma(1+\alpha)} \frac{\Delta}{T^{1-\alpha}}, \quad \Delta \ll T, \tag{21}$$

which shows a clear disparity with the ensemble averaged MSD (5). Despite the anomalous nature of the process, the dependence of the time averaged MSD (21) on the lag time Δ is the same as for Brownian motion. Only the fact that the amplitude decays as function of the measurement time T reflects the anomaly: while the process evolves in time, increasingly longer individual waiting times occur and cause a decay of the effective diffusivity $\simeq K_\alpha/T^{1-\alpha}$. This behaviour also leads to severe changes in the interaction of a particle with a reactive surface[50,51] and the exploration of phase scape.[52]

Figure 3 shows the time averaged MSD for individual realisations of a subdiffusive CTRW with $\alpha = 0.5$. We notice a distinct scatter of the amplitudes between the realisations. Moreover, while for most realisations the predicted linear slope $\left\langle \overline{\delta^2(\Delta)} \right\rangle \simeq \Delta$ is observed, some of the time traces also show variations in the local slope. Such amplitude scatter and local slope variations are a common feature in many experiments, compare Refs. 17, 18, 45, 53. We can quantify the amplitude scatter in terms of the dimensionless ratio $\xi = \overline{\delta^2(\Delta)} / \left\langle \overline{\delta^2(\Delta)} \right\rangle$. The corresponding distribution of relative amplitudes, $\phi_\alpha(\xi)$ in the case of the subdiffusive CTRW becomes a one-sided Lévy stable distribution.[9,48] This distribution for the limit

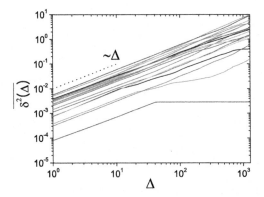

Fig. 3. (Color online) Individual trajectories of a scale-free, subdiffusive CTRW with $\alpha = 0.5$ exhibit the linear lag time dependence predicted by Eq. (21), with smaller local variations of the slope. In addition, there is a clear scatter of the amplitudes between individual trajectories. These features reflect the influence of individual long waiting time events.

$T \to \infty$ demonstrates that no matter how long we average the motion of the particle, on the single trajectory level the time averaged MSD of this process always remains a random quantity. In the special case $\alpha = 1/2$ we find the Gaussian form

$$\phi_{1/2}(\xi) = \frac{2}{\pi} \exp\left(-\frac{\xi^2}{\pi}\right). \tag{22}$$

Its maximum is at $\xi = 0$, reflecting completely stalled trajectories during the measurement time T. Mobile trajectories with $\xi > 0$ are distributed as a half Gaussian. When α increases towards the Brownian value $\alpha = 1$, a peak emerges at $\xi = 1$. In the Brownian case $\alpha = 1$, ergodicity is restored, and $\phi_1(\xi) = \delta(\xi - 1)$ indicates that for sufficiently long trajectories each realisation is fully reproducible. This behaviour in terms of $\phi(\xi)$ is independent of an external potential,[54,55] due to the fact that the ratio $\overline{\delta^2(\Delta)} \big/ \left\langle \overline{\delta^2(\Delta)} \right\rangle$ is equal to the ratio $n(T)/\langle n(T) \rangle$ of the number of jumps.[38]

Under confinement, for instance, by an harmonic external potential within a finite domain with reflecting walls, the time averaged MSD of subdiffusive CTRWs does not converge to the thermal plateau of the ensemble averaged MSD. Instead, the time averaged MSD scales like[55,56]

$$\left\langle \overline{\delta^2(\Delta)} \right\rangle \sim \left(\langle x^2 \rangle_B - \langle x \rangle_B^2 \right) \frac{2\sin(\pi\alpha)}{(1-\alpha)\pi\alpha} \left(\frac{\Delta}{T}\right)^{1-\alpha} \tag{23}$$

for $\Delta \ll T$ and $\Delta \gg (1/[K_\alpha \lambda_1])^{1/\alpha}$. λ_1 represents the lowest non-zero eigenvalue of the Fokker-Planck operator in the confining potential, a measure for the time scale when the particle engages with the confinement. The result (23) is universal in so far as only the prefactor depends on the very form of the confining potential $V(x)$. It involves the first and second moments of the Boltzmann distribution, $\langle x^j \rangle_B = \int x^j \exp(-V(x)/[k_B \mathscr{T}])dx/\mathscr{Z}$. The normalisation factor is the partition $\mathscr{Z} = \int \exp(-V(x)/[k_B \mathscr{T}])dx$. The analysis shows that in this scale free process weak non-ergodicity remains present even in the limit of long measurements.

3.1. *Ageing behaviour of subdiffusive CTRW processes*

CTRW processes with diverging time scale display ageing effects.[57,58] We already saw ageing in the presence of the measurement time T in the time averaged MSD (21). Ageing is due to the non-stationarity of the process. Thus, in subdiffusive CTRWs the two-point correlation $\langle x(t_1)x(t_2)\rangle = f(t_1/t_2)$ is not a function of the difference $|t_2 - t_1|$ of the two times but their ratio.[55] This breakdown of stationarity removes the time translation invariance of stationary processes and needs to be taken into consideration in experiments, in which the start of the recording of the trajectories occurs only at some (ageing) time $t_a > 0$ after the original initialisation of the system dynamics at $t = 0$.

For the regular MSD, for sufficiently long ageing times t_a this leads to a crossover from the scaling $\langle x^2(t)\rangle \simeq K_\alpha t/t_a^{1-\alpha}$ in the ageing-dominated regime $t \ll t_a$ to the scaling (5) when the system evolves for much longer than the ageing time, $t \gg t_a$.[38,58] In the same situation the time averaged MSD (15) behaves much simpler and features the multiplicative, universal correction factor[38]

$$\Lambda_\alpha(t_a/T) = \left(1 + \frac{t_a}{T}\right)^\alpha - \left(\frac{t_a}{T}\right)^\alpha. \tag{24}$$

This factor solely depends on the ratio t_a/T of ageing time t_a and measurement time T. Thus, apart from the amplitude, the scaling of the time averaged MSD (15) as function of the lag time Δ remains unaffected, an important piece of knowledge when the exact age t_a of the process is not precisely known.[38]

Ageing of a subdiffusive CTRW process gives rise to another remarkable feature. Namely, the probability to observe at least one jump in an aged trajectory of length T decreases algebraically with the ageing time t_a.[38] This property of the *population splitting* of particles into a mobile and a fully immobile fraction has to be taken into account when we want to deduce the anomalous diffusion constant from aged trajectories.[38] We note that also the first passage time behaviour of aged CTRW processes exhibits an explicit dependence on the ageing time t_a. In particular, interesting crossovers between different scaling regimes occur, a fact that may be used to deduce the age t_a of a system from sufficiently long first passage data.[59]

More specifically, in an aged system the start of the measurement at t_a typically finds the system during one of the long waiting time events. It can be shown that the occurrence of the first jump event in this case at the so-called forward waiting time t_1 is distributed according to,[60–62]

$$\psi_1(t_1|t_a) = \frac{\sin(\pi\alpha)}{\pi} \frac{t_a^\alpha}{t_1^\alpha(t_a + t_1)}. \tag{25}$$

At long waiting times $t_a \gg t_1$ the distribution of the forward waiting time is thus broader than the regular waiting times t in $\psi(t)$. In an aged CTRW all subsequent jumps then follow the law $\psi(t)$ again. Still, due to the macroscopic memory inherent in CTRW processes,[10] the influence of the ageing time persists until the evolution is much longer than t_a. In a modified CTRW model, in which *every* jump is dominated by the forward waiting time (25), the dynamics of the process is significantly slowed down, giving rise to logarithmic time evolutions.[63] These can be connected to single file systems in which each particle separately becomes trapped with a scale-free distribution of trapping times $\psi(t)$.[64]

4. Correlated Continuous Time Random Walks

What if we do away with the renewal property of the previously discussed CTRW process? One way to include correlations into the CTRW process is to consider a model when successive waiting times are only separated by an incremental change. Physically, this could reflect the motion in a quenched environment, in which locally the motion is dominated by a given mobility with small variations. We could thus imagine that the current waiting τ_i is composed of increments in the form[65–67]

$$\tau_i = \left| \xi_1 + \xi_2 + \ldots + \xi_{i-1} \right|. \tag{26}$$

If the ξ_i are distributed according to a Lévy stable law defined in terms of its Fourier transform $\exp\left(-c_\gamma |k|^\gamma\right)$ with $0 < \gamma < 2$, then the process leads to anomalous diffusion governed by Eq. (5) with the anomalous diffusion exponent $\alpha = \gamma/(1+\gamma)$. Its range is $0 < \alpha < 2/3$.[65,66] This model features a stretched exponential mode relaxation $P(k,t) \simeq \exp(-ct^{1/2})$ in the limit $\gamma = 2$, while for for $0 < \gamma < 2$ a power-law form $P(k,t) \simeq t^{-\gamma}$ is obtained.[67] There also exist alternative models to correlated jump processes, see the discussion in Refs. 68 and 69 and the citations therein.

The absolute value in the law (26) implies that the mean waiting time keeps growing with T and diverges in the long time limit. The time averaged MSD[67]

$$\left\langle \overline{\delta^2(\Delta)} \right\rangle \simeq \frac{\Delta}{T^{1-\gamma/(1+\gamma)}} \tag{27}$$

shows the weakly non-ergodic behaviour of the correlated CTRW process. It also features ageing effects demonstrated by the temporal decay of the response of the system to a periodic driving force.[67] Individual trajectories show a pronounced amplitude scatter.[65]

A similar trick can be used to correlate subsequent jump lengths. The MSD of this process is then given exactly by[65]

$$\langle x(t)^2 \rangle \simeq \frac{t(t+1)(2t+1)\sigma^2}{4}, \tag{28}$$

for a Gaussian distribution of jump increments with variance σ^2. This process thus has the cubic long time scaling behaviour $\langle x(t)^2 \rangle \simeq t^3$. The associated time averaged MSD scales quadratically,[65]

$$\left\langle \overline{\delta^2(\Delta)} \right\rangle \simeq \Delta^2 T \tag{29}$$

for $\Delta \ll T$. Thus, also this process is weakly non-ergodic.[65]

5. Heterogeneous Diffusion Processes

Let us now address a seemingly much simpler scenario, namely, a diffusion process with a space-dependent diffusivity $K(x)$. Such descriptions were used to model turbulence[70] or diffusion in heterogenous porous media.[71,72] In biological cells, local variations of the diffusion coefficient were indeed recently mapped out.[73] We consider the Langevin equation[74]

$$\frac{dx(t)}{dt} = \sqrt{2K(x)} \times \xi(t), \tag{30}$$

where the multiplicative noise $\xi(t)$ is white and Gaussian with zero mean. Using the Stratonovich interpretation this heterogeneous diffusion process (HDP) can be shown to be weakly non-ergodic.

Consider the power-law form $K(x) \simeq K_0|x|^\beta$ for the diffusivity. The MSD is then given by[74]

$$\langle x^2(t) \rangle = \frac{\Gamma(p + 1/2)}{\pi^{1/2}} \left(\frac{2}{p}\right)^{2p} (K_0 t)^p, \tag{31}$$

with the exponent $p = 2/(2 - \beta)$. For $\beta < 0$ this process is therefore subdiffusive, while for $0 < \beta < 2$ it is superdiffusive.[74] The time averaged MSD in the limit $\Delta \ll T$ exhibits the linear dependence[74]

$$\left\langle \overline{\delta^2(\Delta)} \right\rangle = \frac{\Gamma(p + 1/2)}{\pi^{1/2}} \left(\frac{2}{p}\right)^{2p} K_0^p \frac{\Delta}{T^{1-p}} \tag{32}$$

on the lag time, valid for both sub- and superdiffusive regimes. This implies the exact connection $\langle \overline{\delta^2(\Delta)} \rangle = (\Delta/T)^{1-p}\langle x^2(\Delta) \rangle$ with the ensemble averaged MSD.

Interestingly, despite the simplicity of the HDP process we again observe a weakly non-ergodic behaviour. Similar results follow in the case of fast (exponential) and slow (logarithmic) variations of the diffusivity $K(x)$ with the particle position x.[75] We note that for the exponential case the square root scaling $\langle \overline{\delta^2(\Delta)} \rangle \simeq \Delta^{1/2}$ was observed.[75] In the context of imaged diffusion in cells the HDP process with power-law x-dependence of $K(x)$ was also generalised to two dimensions.[76]

6. Scaled Brownian Motion

What if we consider a time-dependent diffusion coefficient instead of the x-dependence? As pointed out by Fuliński already,[77] such experimentally observed variations of the diffusivity[78] may cause weakly non-ergodic behaviour in analogy to the spatial dependence in the HDP process above. For a power-law time dependence of the diffusivity this process is so-called scaled Brownian motion (SBM).[79] Let us start with the Langevin equation

$$\frac{dx(t)}{dt} = \sqrt{2\mathscr{K}(t)} \times \xi(t), \tag{33}$$

where $\xi(t)$ is white Gaussian noise with zero mean. The diffusion coefficient is given by

$$\mathcal{K}(t) = \alpha K_\alpha t^{\alpha-1}, \tag{34}$$

where $0 < \alpha < 2$. This process obviously leads to the MSD (5). Concurrently, the time averaged MSD has the exact form[80]

$$\left\langle \overline{\delta^2(\Delta)} \right\rangle = \frac{2K_\alpha t^{1+\alpha}}{(\alpha+1)} \frac{\left[1 - (\Delta/T)^{1+\alpha} - (1 - \Delta/T)^{1+\alpha}\right]}{T - \Delta}. \tag{35}$$

For $\Delta \ll T$, the linear Δ-scaling is recovered,[81]

$$\left\langle \overline{\delta^2(\Delta)} \right\rangle \sim 2K_\alpha \frac{\Delta}{T^{1-\alpha}} \tag{36}$$

in both the sub- and superdiffusive cases. Thus, again we obtain a weakly non-ergodic behaviour given by the disparity between ensemble and time averaged MSD. However, different to the above weakly non-ergodic processes, SBM features fully reproducible trajectories in the long time limit.[80,81] As discussed in Ref. 80 in detail, the time dependent diffusivity $\mathcal{K}(t)$ may appear as a simple and natural choice for the description of anomalous diffusion processes. However, $\mathcal{K}(t)$ actually reflects a time-dependent temperature,[77,80] and thus leads to unphysical behaviour in thermalised systems, in particular, when the data are from a confined system, for instance, when the trajectories are measured by optical tweezers methods.[80]

7. Conclusions

Single particle tracking is increasingly becoming a standard tool to study the motion of tracer particles in systems such as complex fluids or even living biological cells. Concurrently, single particle traces are evaluated in large scale computer simulations, for instance, to detect inhomogeneous motion in a population of simulated particles. To evaluate the garnered time series one typically uses the time averaged MSD. As we showed here, when the motion of the particle is anomalous, care has to be taken to evaluate the results in a physically meaningful way. Due to the occurrence of transient or asymptotic weak ergodicity breaking, one cannot simply compare the results for the time averages with the known behaviour of the corresponding ensemble averages.

Apart from the processes discussed herein, non-ergodic behaviour also occurs in other stochastic processes, including the ultraweakly non-ergodic Lévy walks[82–84] where the disparity between ensemble and time averaged MSDs only amounts to a constant factor. Diffusion on random, fractal percolation clusters was shown to be ergodic.[85] We also note that in some systems combinations of stochastic processes have to be applied to capture the observed data.[17,18,45,86–88]

The diagnosis of a given data set for the exact underlying stochastic process[11–14] requires the analysis of several complementary quantities. We mention the amplitude scatter statistics,[29] increment autocorrelations,[9, 23] higher order moments,[89, 90] mean maximal excursion methods,[89] p-variation,[91, 92] and the analysis of the distribution of the apparent diffusivity.[93]

Acknowledgments

The author acknowledges funding from the Academy of Finland within the Finland Distinguished Professor scheme.

References

1. R. Brown, Phil. Mag. **4**, 161, 1828.
2. A. Einstein, Ann. d. Physik **17**, 549 (1905).
3. M. von Smoluchowsky, Ann. Phys. (Leipzig) **21**, 756 (1906).
4. P. Langevin, C. R. Acad. Sci. Paris **146**, 530 (1908).
5. J. Perrin, C. R. Acad. Sci. Paris **146**, 967 (1908).
6. I. Nordlund, Z. Phys. Chem. **87**, 40 (1914).
7. E. Kappler, Ann. d. Phys. (Leipzig) **11**, 233 (1931).
8. C. Bräuchle, D. C. Lamb, and J. Michaelis, Single Particle Tracking and Single Molecule Energy Transfer (Wiley-VCH, Weinheim, Germany, 2012); X. S. Xie, P. J. Choi, G.-W. Li, N. K. Lee, and G. Lia, Annu. Rev. Biophys. **37**, 417 (2008).
9. S. Burov, J.-H. Jeon, R. Metzler, and E. Barkai, Phys. Chem. Chem. Phys. **13**, 1800 (2011).
10. R. Metzler and J. Klafter, Phys. Rep. **339**, 1 (2000); J. Phys. A **37**, R161 (2004).
11. M. J. Saxton and K. Jacobson, Annu. Rev. Biophys. Biomol. Struct. **26**, 373 (1997).
12. E. Barkai, Y. Garini, and R. Metzler, Physics Today **65**(8), 29 (2012).
13. F. Höfling and T. Franosch, Rep. Prog. Phys. **76**, 046602 (2013).
14. I. M. Sokolov, Soft Matter **8**, 9043 (2012).
15. W. T. Coffey and Yu. P. Kalmykov, The Langevin Equation: With Applications to Stochastic Problems in Physics, Chemistry and Electrical Engineering (World Scientific, Singapore, 2012).
16. I. Goychuk, Phys. Rev. E **80**, 046125 (2009); Adv. Chem. Phys. **150**, 187 (2012).
17. J.-H. Jeon, V. Tejedor, S. Burov, E. Barkai, C. Selhuber-Unkel, K. Berg-Sørensen, L. Oddershede, and R. Metzler, Phys. Rev. Lett. **106**, 048103 (2011).
18. S. M. A. Tabei, S. Burov, H. Y. Kim, A. Kuznetsov, T. Huynh, J. Jureller, L. H. Philipson, A. R. Dinner, and N. F. Scherer, Proc. Natl. Acad. Sci. USA **110**, 4911 (2013).
19. J.-H. Jeon, N. Leijnse, L. B. Oddershede, and R. Metzler, New J. Phys. **15**, 045011 (2013).
20. S. C. Weber, A. J. Spakowitz, and J. A. Theriot, Phys. Rev. Lett. **104**, 238102 (2010).
21. J. Szymanski and M. Weiss, Phys. Rev. Lett. **103**, 038102 (2009).
22. G. R. Kneller, K. Baczynski, and M. Pasenkiewicz-Gierula, J. Chem. Phys. **135**, 141105 (2011).
23. J.-H. Jeon, H. Martinez-Seara Monne, M. Javanainen, and R. Metzler, Phys. Rev. Lett. **109**, 188103 (2012).
24. M. Javanainen, H. Hammaren, L. Monticelli, J.-H. Jeon, R. Metzler, and I. Vattulainen, Faraday Disc. **161**, 397 (2013).

25. T. E. Harris, J. Appl. Prob. **2**(2), 323 (1965).
26. A. N. Kolmogorov, Dokl. Acad. Sci. USSR **26**, 115 (1940).
27. B. B. Mandelbrot and J. W. van Ness, SIAM Rev. **1**, 422 (1968).
28. W. Deng and E. Barkai, Phys. Rev. E **79**, 011112 (2009).
29. J.-H. Jeon and R. Metzler, J. Phys. A **43**, 252001 (2010).
30. R. Zwanzig, Nonequilibrium Statistical Mechanics (Oxford University Press, Oxford, UK, 2001).
31. F. Mainardi, Fractional calculus and waves in linear viscoelasticity (Imperial College Press, London, 2010).
32. E. Lutz, Phys. Rev. E **64**, 051106 (2001).
33. I. Goychuk, V. O. Kharchenko, and R. Metzler, PLoS ONE **9**, e91700 (2014); Phys. Chem. Chem. Phys. DOI: 10.1039/C4CP01234H.
34. J.-H. Jeon and R. Metzler, Phys. Rev. E **81**, 021103 (2010).
35. O. Yu. Sliusarenko, V. Yu. Gonchar, A. V. Chechkin, I. M. Sokolov, and R. Metzler, Phys. Rev. E **81**, 041119 (2010).
36. J.-H. Jeon and R. Metzler, Phys. Rev. E **85**, 021147 (2012).
37. J. Kursawe, J. H. P. Schulz, and R. Metzler, Phys. Rev. E **88**, 062124 (2013).
38. J. H. P. Schulz, E. Barkai, and R. Metzler, Phys. Rev. Lett. **110**, 020602 (2013); Phys. Rev. X **4**, 011028 (2014).
39. E. W. Montroll and G. H. Weiss, J. Math. Phys. **6**, 167 (1965).
40. H. Scher and E. W. Montroll, Phys. Rev. B **12**, 2455 (1975).
41. B. D. Hughes, Random Walks and Random Environments, Volume 1: Random Walks (Oxford University Press, Oxford, 1995).
42. H. Scher, G. Margolin, R. Metzler, J. Klafter, and B. Berkowitz, Geophys. Res. Lett. **29**, 1061 (2002).
43. I. Y. Wong, M. L. Gardel, D. R. Reichman, E. R. Weeks, M. T. Valentine, A. R. Bausch, and D. A. Weitz, Phys. Rev. Lett. **92**, 178101 (2004).
44. Q. Xu, L. Feng, R. Sha, N. C. Seeman, and P. M. Chaikin, Phys. Rev. Lett. **106**, 228102 (2011).
45. A. V. Weigel, B. Simon, M. M. Tamkun, and D. Krapf, Proc. Nat. Acad. Sci. USA **108**, 6438 (2011).
46. J.-P. Bouchaud, J. Phys. I **2**, 1705 (1992).
47. G. Bel and E. Barkai, Phys. Rev. Lett. **94**, 240602 (2005).
48. Y. He, S. Burov, R. Metzler, and E. Barkai, Phys. Rev. Lett. **101**, 058101 (2008).
49. A. Lubelski, I. M. Sokolov, and J. Klafter, Phys. Rev. Lett. **100**, 250602 (2008).
50. M. A. Lomholt, I. M. Zaid, and R. Metzler, Phys. Rev. Lett. **98**, 200603 (2007); I. M. Zaid, M. A. Lomholt, and R. Metzler, Biophys. J. **97**, 710 (2009).
51. M. J. Skaug, A. M. Lacasta, L. Ramirez-Piscina, J. M. Sancho, K. Lindenberg, and D. K. Schwartz, Soft Matter **10**, 753 (2014); M. Khoury, A. M. Lacasta, J. M. Sancho, and K. Lindenberg, Phys. Rev. Lett. **106**, 090602 (2011).
52. G. Bel and E. Barkai, J. Phys. Cond. Mat. **17**, S4287 (2005); Phys. Rev. Lett. **94**, 240602 (2005); A. Rebenshtok and E. Barkai, J. Stat. Phys. **133**, 565 (2008); Phys. Rev. Lett. **99**, 210601 (2007).
53. I. Golding and E. C. Cox, Phys. Rev. Lett. **96**, 098102 (2006).
54. I. M. Sokolov, E. Heinsalu, P. Hänggi and I. Goychuk, Europhys. Lett. **86**, 30009 (2009).
55. S. Burov, R. Metzler, and E. Barkai, Proc. Natl. Acad. Sci. USA **107**, 13228 (2010).
56. T. Neusius, I. M. Sokolov, and J. C. Smith, Phys. Rev. E **80**, 011109 (2009).
57. C. Monthus and J.-P. Bouchaud, J. Phys. A *29*, 3847 (1996).
58. E. Barkai and Y. C. Cheng, J. Chem. Phys. **118**, 6167 (2003).

59. H. Krüsemann, A. Godec, and R. Metzler, Phys. Rev. E **89**, 040101(R) (2014).
60. E. B. Dynkin, Izv. Akad. Nauk. SSSR Ser. Math. **19**, 247 (1955); Selected Translations Math. Stat. Prob. **1**, 171 (1961).
61. C. Godrèche and J. M. Luck, J. Stat. Phys. **104**, 489 (2001); E. Barkai and Y.-C. Cheng, J. Chem. Phys. **118**, 6167 (2003); E. Barkai, Phys. Rev. Lett. **90**, 104101 (2003).
62. T. Koren, M. A. Lomholt, A. V. Chechkin, J. Klafter, and R. Metzler, Phys. Rev. Lett. **99**, 160602 (2007).
63. M. A. Lomholt, L. Lizana, R. Metzler, and T. Ambjörnsson, Phys. Rev. Lett. **110**, 208301 (2013).
64. L. P. Sanders, M. A. Lomholt, L. Lizana, K. Fogelmark, R. Metzler, and T. Ambjörnsson, E-print arXiv:1311.3790.
65. V. Tejedor and R. Metzler, J. Phys. A **43**, 082002 (2010).
66. M. Magdziarz, R. Metzler, W. Szczotka, and P. Zebrowski, Phys. Rev. E **85**, 051103 (2012).
67. M. Magdziarz, R. Metzler, W. Szczotka, and P. Zebrowski, J. Stat. Mech. P04010 (2012).
68. A. V. Chechkin, M. Hofmann, and I. M. Sokolov, Phys. Rev. E **80**, 031112 (2009).
69. J. H. P. Schulz, A. V. Chechkin, and R. Metzler, J. Phys. A. **46**, 475001 (2013).
70. L. F. Richardson, Proc. Roy. Soc. London, Ser. A **110**, 709 (1926); A. S. Monin and A. M. Yaglom, Statistical Fluid Mechanics (MIT Press, Cambdridge MA, 1971).
71. M. Dentz, P. Gouze, A. Russian, J. Dweik, and F. Delay, Adv. Water Res. **49**, 13 (2012).
72. C. Loverdo et al., Phys. Rev. Lett. **102**, 188101 (2009).
73. T. Kühn, T. O. Ihalainen, J. Hyväluoma, N. Dross, S. F. Willman, J. Langowski, M. Vihinen-Ranta, and J. Timonen, PLoS One **6**, e22962 (2011).
74. A. G. Cherstvy, A. V. Chechkin, and R. Metzler, New J. Phys. **15**, 083039 (2013).
75. A. G. Cherstvy and R. Metzler, Phys. Chem. Chem. Phys. **15**, 20220 (2013).
76. A. V. Cherstvy, A. V. Chechkin, and R. Metzler, Soft Matter **10**, 1591 (2014).
77. A. Fuliński, Phys. Rev. E **83**, 061140 (2011); J. Chem. Phys. **138**, 021101 (2013).
78. M. Platani, I. Goldberg, A. I. Lamond, and J. R. Swedlow, Nature Cell Biol. **4**, 502 (2002).
79. S. C. Lim and S. V. Muniandy, Phys. Rev. E **66**, 021114 (2002).
80. J.-H. Jeon, A. V. Chechkin, and R. Metzler, Phys. Chem. Chem. Phys. DOI: 10.1039/c4cp02019g.
81. F. Thiel and I. M. Sokolov, Phys. Rev. E **89**, 012115 (2014).
82. G. Zumofen and J. Klafter, Physica D **69**, 436 (1993).
83. A. Godec and R. Metzler, Phys. Rev. Lett. **110**, 020603 (2013); Phys. Rev. E **88**, 012116 (2013).
84. D. Froemberg and E. Barkai, Phys. Rev. E **87**, 030104(R) (2013); Phys. Rev. E **88**, 024101 (2013).
85. Y. Meroz, I. Eliazar, and J. Klafter, J. Phys. A **42**, 434012 (2009); Y. Meroz, I. M. Sokolov, and J. Klafter, Phys. Rev. Lett. **110**, 090601 (2013).
86. T. Akimoto, E. Yamamoto, K. Yasuoka, Y. Hirano, and M. Yasui, Phys. Rev. Lett. **107**, 178103 (2011).
87. J.-H. Jeon, E. Barkai, and R. Metzler, J. Chem. Phys. **139**, 121916 (2013).
88. S. Eule and R. Friedrich, Phys. Rev. E **87**, 032162 (2013).
89. V. Tejedor, O. Bénichou, R. Voituriez, R. Jungmann, F. Simmel, C. Selhuber-Unkel, L. Oddershede, and R. Metzler, Biophys. J. **98**, 1364 (2010).
90. D. Ernst, J. Kohler, and M. Weiss, Phys. Chem. Chem. Phys. **16**, 7686 (2014).

91. M. Magdziarz, A. Weron, K. Burnecki, and J. Klafter, Phys. Rev. Lett. **103**, 180602 (2009)
92. K. Burnecki, E. Kepten, J. Janczura, I. Bronshtein, Y. Garini, and A. Weron, Biophys. J. **103**, 1839 (2012).
93. M. Bauer, R. Valiullin, G. Radons, and J. Kaerger, J. Chem. Phys. **135**, 144118 (2011).

7th Jagna International Workshop (2014)
International Journal of Modern Physics: Conference Series
Vol. 36 (2015) 1560008 (16 pages)
© The Authors
DOI: 10.1142/S2010194515600083

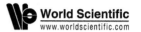
World Scientific
www.worldscientific.com

Fractional dispersive transport in inhomogeneous organic semiconductors

K. Y. Choo* and S. V. Muniandy†

*Department of Physics, University of Malaya,
50603, Kuala Lumpur, Malaysia*
†*msithi@um.edu.my*
http://fizik.um.edu.my/svm/Profile.html

Published 2 January 2015

The study of transport dynamics of charge carriers in homogeneous and inhomogeneous organic semiconductor using the variable order time-fractional drift-diffusion equation (VO-TFDDE) is presented in this paper. The fractional-time derivative operator and spatial derivative operator of the time-fractional drift-diffusion equation are discretized respectively using the implicit difference scheme and the centered difference scheme. Self-consistent Poisson solver was incorporated in the model to solve for the electric potential and the localized electric field that sweeps the charge carriers across the device. The homogeneity of the material is represented by the different values or functions of the fractional derivative order. Diffusion transport dynamics is observed when charge carriers are moving in homogeneous crystalline-like structure. In contrast, dispersive transport dynamics is observed when charge carriers are moving in homogeneous amorphous-like structure. For inhomogeneous amorphous-crystalline-mixed structure, pulse broadening effect is impeded as charge carriers are moving towards the crystalline-like region at the other end of the device. Conversely, pulse broadening effect is getting severe if charge carriers are moving across the device with inhomogeneous crystalline-amorphous-mixed structure. Therefore, in order to achieve diffusive-like transport dynamics that could reduce the pulse broadening effect, homogeneous crystalline-like structure or inhomogeneous amorphous-crystalline-mixed structure is recommended for device fabrication.

Keywords: Fractional diffusion equation; dispersive transport; organic semiconductor.

1. Introduction

The discovery of conducting polymer, polyacetylene doped with halogens in 1977 by Heeger, MacDiarmid and Shirakawa has triggered tremendous research in organic electronic materials[1]. Extensive collaborative efforts among physicists, chemists,

---

*The author is also affiliated to the Faculty of Engineering, Multimedia University, Jalan Multimedia, 63100 Cyberjaya, Selangor D.E., Malaysia. Email: kychoo@mmu.edu.my

material scientists and device engineers were mobilized to study the electrical, optical, thermal and mechanical properties of organic or polymer materials. In addition, low-cost, low-temperature and simpler fabrication processes involved in the fabrication of an organic material, and its elasticity property, have further made organic material as the promising material for making various types of electronic and opto-electronic devices. Some of the popular organic-based devices are organic solar cells[2], organic light emitting diodes[3], and organic field-effect transistors[4]. Unfortunately, the low carrier mobility, low thermal tolerance and performance degradation due to oxidation of organic materials have hindered the application of organic materials in high-speed, high-temperature and high-power applications. Particularly, the low carrier mobility suffered by organic materials broadens the pulse width of the electrical-injected or photo-generated current pulse in the device. This further reduces the speed performance of the device in responding to a pulse train with high-repetition rate. Numerous kinetic theories have been proposed to explain the possible physical mechanisms that govern the pulse broadening effect of the current pulse such as the multiple trapping mechanism due to exponential energy distribution of the localized states and charge carrier conduction via hopping mechanism[5-7].

The observation of the universality of long-tail behaviour of transient photocurrent in a disorder semiconductor obtained from the time-of-flight measurement suggests that the transport dynamics could be studied through Brownian motion or its generalizations. One of the charge carrier transport frameworks is the continuous time random walk (CTRW) model proposed by Schear and Montrell[5]. In the CTRW framework, the dispersive transport due to the multiple trapping time mechanism is described by writing the hopping time distribution as in the power-law form of $\psi(t) \sim t^{1+\alpha}$ where $0 < \alpha < 1$, with the asymptotic property used to account for the long-tail behaviour of the transient photocurrent observed in disorder semiconductor material. The scaling parameter α is useful to deduce the type of the transport dynamics of the charge carriers. For example, exponent $\alpha \neq 1$ gives the sub-diffusion type process while $\alpha = 1$ represents the standard diffusion process.

The long-tail behaviour of transient photocurrent observed in disorder semiconductor also implied that the transport dynamics in disorder semiconductor deviates from the standard kinetic transport model that is derived based on the Fick's law. Thus, various types of kinetic transport models have been established to study the dispersive transport of charge carriers in disorder semiconductor. These models include the fractional Fokker-Planck equation[8-11], fractional differential approach consisting of various forms of fractional drift-diffusion equations[12-13], fractional Langevin equation[14-15], fractional Klein-Kramer equation[16], Levy-space-fractional diffusion equation[17-18] and Levy-space-fractional Fokker-Planck equation[19].

In this work, we study how the transport dynamics of charge carriers is influenced by the homogeneity and inhomogeneity of the organic semiconductor using the variable-order time-fractional drift-diffusion equation (VOTFDDE). The numerical scheme previously developed to solve the time-fractional diffusion equation[20-21] was employed here to solve the VOTFDDE. Section 2 presents the mathematical background used to describe the dispersive transport dynamics of charge carrier in homogeneous and inhomogeneous organic semiconductor. The procedures of solving the VOTFDDE, self-consistent Poisson solver and current density are outlined in Section 3. Discussion of the simulated results are given in Section 4 and followed by the conclusion in Section 5.

2. Mathematical Modeling of Dispersive Transport

2.1. *Variable order time-fractional drift-diffusion equation*

The standard one-dimensional diffusion equation (DE) used to model charge carrier transport dynamics in non-disorder material such as a crystalline semiconductor is given as

$$\frac{\partial n(x,t)}{\partial t} = D\frac{\partial^2 n(x,t)}{\partial x^2}, \tag{1}$$

where $n(x,t)$ is the charge carrier density and D is diffusion constant. If the material is subjected to an external perturbation such as an electric field, a charge carrier will be forced to drift either parallel or anti-parallel with the direction of the electric field. Thus, the standard one-dimensional drift-diffusion equation (DDE) is rewritten based on Eq. (1) as

$$\frac{\partial n(x,t)}{\partial t} = D\frac{\partial^2 n(x,t)}{\partial x^2} - v(x,t)\frac{\partial n(x,t)}{\partial x}, \tag{2}$$

where the velocity of the charge carrier is

$$v(x,t) = \mu E(x,t), \tag{3}$$

μ is its mobility and $E(x,t)$ is the localized electric field.

However, Eq. (1) and Eq. (2) are not adequate to model the charge carrier transport dynamics in disorder material such as amorphous semiconductor and organic semiconductor. This is because the charge carrier diffuses with highly fluctuating diffusivity that results in dispersive transport which is a complex process consisting of various Gaussian processes with wide distribution of their statistical parameters. The dispersive transport causes the transient photocurrent distribution measured from the disorder semiconductor material having an asymptotic power-law behavior with a distribution of the scaling exponent[22] $\alpha(x,t)$. Therefore, the one-dimensional diffusion equation in Eq. (1) and the one-dimensional drift-diffusion equation in Eq. (2) can be generalized to represent the dispersive transport by taking the variable order fractional-time derivative on Eq. (1) and Eq. (2). The variable order one-dimensional time-fractional diffusion equation[20–21] (VOTFDE) and the variable order one-dimensional time-fractional drift-diffusion equation (VOTFDDE) are rewritten respectively as

$$\frac{\partial^{\alpha(x,t)} n(x,t)}{\partial t^{\alpha(x,t)}} = D\frac{\partial^2 n(x,t)}{\partial x^2}, \tag{4}$$

and

$$\frac{\partial^{\alpha(x,t)} n\left(x,t\right)}{\partial t^{\alpha(x,t)}} = D\frac{\partial^2 n\left(x,t\right)}{\partial x^2} - v\left(x,t\right)\frac{\partial n\left(x,t\right)}{\partial x}, \tag{5}$$

where the $\alpha(x,t)$ is the variable order fractional derivative order which can be expressed as a function of time, space or independent variables. If $\alpha(x,t) = 1$, Eq. (4) and Eq. (5) reduce to the standard diffusion equation and standard drift-diffusion equation as shown in Eq. (1) and Eq. (2). The variable order (VO) time-fractional derivative is expressed using the Caputo fractional derivative definition as

$$\frac{\partial^{\alpha(x,t)} n\left(x,t\right)}{\partial t^{\alpha(x,t)}} = \frac{1}{\Gamma\left(1-\alpha\left(x,t\right)\right)}\int_0^t \frac{\partial n\left(x,s\right)}{\partial s}\frac{ds}{\left(t-s\right)^{\alpha(x,t)}}, \quad 0 < \alpha\left(x,t\right) \le 1. \tag{6}$$

Owing to the difficulty in discretization of the time-fractional derivative, the Caputo derivative is usually expressed in terms of the Riemann-Liouville fractional derivative and then approximated using Grüwald-Letnikov derivative to obtain the solution[23]. Nevertheless, Lin and Xu[20] and Sun *et al.*[21] had demonstrated a finite difference scheme to discretize the Caputo time-fractional derivative and were able to obtain the solution for the time-fractional diffusion equation.

2.2. Electric potential and electric field

The electric potential $V(x,t)$ established in the material is obtained by solving the self-consistent Poisson equation consisting of the charge carrier density,

$$\frac{\partial^2 V\left(x,t\right)}{\partial x^2} = -\frac{\rho\left(x,t\right)}{\varepsilon} = -\frac{en\left(x,t\right)}{\varepsilon_r \varepsilon_0}, \tag{7}$$

where $\rho(x,t)$ is the charge density, e is the value of the electronic charge, ε_r is the relative permittivity of the material and ε_0 is the permittivity of vacuum. The localized electric field in Eq. (3) is then obtained through the following equation as

$$E\left(x,t\right) = -\frac{\partial V\left(x,t\right)}{\partial x}. \tag{8}$$

2.3. Current density

The total current density J_T (for a single type charge carrier) is obtained as the sum of the diffusion current density J_{diff} and drift current density J_{drift} as given below

$$J_T\left(x,t\right) = J_{drift}\left(x,t\right) - J_{diff}\left(x,t\right). \tag{9}$$

$$J_T\left(x,t\right) = en\left(x,t\right)\mu E\left(x,t\right) - eD\frac{\partial n\left(x,t\right)}{\partial x}. \tag{10}$$

3. Numerical Method

3.1. *Numerical scheme for variable order time-fractional drift-diffusion equation*

Owing to the unconditional stability offered by the implicit difference scheme, thus it is used to discretize the Caputo-type variable order fractional-time derivative. Define the following: position is $x_i = i\Delta x$ for $0 \le i \le N_x$, time is $t_k = k\Delta t$ for $0 \le k \le N_t - 1$, spatial step is $\Delta x = L/N_x$, time step is $\Delta t = T/N_t$, T is the total time, L is the device length, N_t is the total time step and N_x is the total spatial step. Equation (6) is approximated as[20–21],

$$\frac{\partial^{\alpha(x_i, t_{k+1})} n(x_i, t_{k+1})}{\partial t^{\alpha(x_i, t_{k+1})}}$$

$$= \frac{1}{\Gamma(1 - \alpha(x_i, t_{k+1}))} \sum_{m=0}^{k} \int_{t_m}^{t_{m+1}} \frac{\partial n(x_i, s)}{\partial s} \frac{ds}{(t_{k+1} - s)^{\alpha(x_i, t_{k+1})}}$$

$$= \frac{1}{\Gamma(1 - \alpha(x_i, t_{k+1}))} \sum_{m=0}^{k} \frac{n(x_i, t_{m+1}) - n(x_i, t_m)}{\Delta t}$$

$$\times \int_{t_m}^{t_{m+1}} \frac{ds}{(t_{k+1} - s)^{\alpha(x_i, t_{k+1})}} + O(\Delta t)$$

$$= \frac{1}{\Gamma(2 - \alpha(x_i, t_{k+1}))} \sum_{m=0}^{k} \frac{n(x_i, t_{k+1-m}) - n(x_i, t_{k-m})}{\Delta t^{\alpha(x_i, t_{n+1})}} b_{i,m}^{k+1} + O(\Delta t)$$

where

$$b_i^{m,k+1} = (m + 1)^{1-\alpha(x_i, t_{k+1})} - m^{1-\alpha(x_i, t_{k+1})}, \quad m = 0, 1, \dots, k, \qquad (11)$$

and $b_0 = 1$, $b_m \to 0$ as $m \to \infty$ and $O(\Delta t)$ is the approximation error. Hence, the discrete variable order time-fractional differential operator is written as

$$L_t^{\alpha(x_i, t_{k+1})} n(x_i, t_{k+1}) := \frac{1}{\Gamma(2 - \alpha(x_i, t_{k+1}))}$$

$$\times \sum_{m=0}^{k} b_i^{m,k+1} \frac{n(x_i, t_{k+1-m}) - n(x_i, t_{k-m})}{\Delta t^{\alpha(x_i, t_{k+1})}}, \qquad (12)$$

and finally Eq. (6) is rewritten as

$$\frac{\partial^{\alpha(x_i, t_{k+1})} n(x_i, t_{k+1})}{\partial t^{\alpha(x_i, t_{k+1})}} = L_t^{\alpha(x_i, t_{k+1})} n(x_i, t_{k+1}) + O(\Delta t). \qquad (13)$$

In order to implement the Caputo fractional derivative, the results of the integer order time-derivative of $n(x,t)$ at all the previous time steps are required.

Apply Eq. (13) and taking the centered difference scheme on the space derivative of Eq. (5), the VOTFDDE is approximated as

$$\frac{\partial^{\alpha(x_i,t_{k+1})} n(x_i,t_{k+1})}{\partial t^{\alpha(x_i,t_{k+1})}} = D\frac{\partial^2 n(x_i,t_{k+1})}{\partial x^2} - v(x_i,t_{k+1})\frac{\partial n(x_i,t_{k+1})}{\partial x}. \tag{14}$$

$$L_t^{\alpha(x_i,t_{k+1})} n(x_i,t_{k+1}) = D\left[\frac{n(x_{i+1},t_{k+1}) - 2n(x_i,t_{k+1}) + n(x_{i-1},t_{k+1})}{(\Delta x)^2}\right]$$
$$-v(x_i,t_{k+1})\left[\frac{n(x_{i+1},t_{k+1}) - n(x_{i-1},t_{k+1})}{2\Delta x}\right] + O\left((\Delta x)^2\right). \tag{15}$$

Let's define

$$n(x_i,t_k) = n(i\Delta x, k\Delta t) = n_i^k, \tag{16}$$

and

$$v(x_i,t_k) = v(i\Delta x, k\Delta t) = v_i^k. \tag{17}$$

Rewriting the VOTFDDE in Eq. (15) by grouping the t_{k+1} terms on the LHS and t_k terms on the RHS, one gets

$$n_i^{k+1} - \frac{D\Gamma\left(2 - \alpha_i^{k+1}\right)\Delta t^{\alpha_i^{k+1}}}{(\Delta x)^2}\left(n_{i+1}^{k+1} - 2n_i^{k+1} + n_{i-1}^{k+1}\right)$$
$$+ \frac{v_i^{k+1}\Gamma\left(2 - \alpha_i^{k+1}\right)\Delta t^{\alpha_i^{k+1}}}{2\Delta x}\left(n_{i+1}^{k+1} - n_{i-1}^{k+1}\right)$$
$$= \left(1 - b_i^{1,k+1}\right)n_i^k + \sum_{m=1}^{k-1}\left(b_i^{m,k+1} - b_i^{m+1,k+1}\right)n_i^{k-m} + b_i^{k,k+1}n_i^0.$$

By defining

$$C_{D,i}^{k+1} = \frac{D\Gamma\left(2 - \alpha_i^{k+1}\right)\Delta t^{\alpha_i^{k+1}}}{(\Delta x)^2} \quad \text{and} \quad C_{v,i}^{k+1} = \frac{v_i^{k+1}\Gamma\left(2 - \alpha_i^{k+1}\right)\Delta t^{\alpha_i^{k+1}}}{2\Delta x}, \tag{18}$$

the VOTFDDE becomes

$$\left(-C_{D,i}^{k+1} - C_{v,i}^{k+1}\right)n_{i-1}^{k+1} + \left(1 + 2C_{D,i}^{k+1}\right)n_i^{k+1} + \left(-C_{D,i}^{k+1} + C_{v,i}^{k+1}\right)n_{i+1}^{k+1}$$
$$= \left(1 - b_i^{1,k+1}\right)n_i^k + \sum_{m=1}^{k-1}\left(b_i^{m,k+1} - b_i^{m+1,k+1}\right)n_i^{k-m} + b_i^{k,k+1}n_i^0, \quad k \geq 1. \tag{19}$$

When $k = 0$ and $\alpha = 1$, Eq. (19) reduces to the standard drift-diffusion equation.

$$\left(-C_{D,i}^1 - C_{v,i}^1\right) n_{i-1}^1 + \left(1 + 2C_{D,i}^1\right) n_i^1 + \left(-C_{D,i}^1 + C_{v,i}^1\right) n_{i+1}^1 = n_i^0, \quad b_i^{0,1} = 1. \quad (20)$$

Eq. (20) can be solved using the matrix method. Define that

$$P_{i-1}^{k+1} = -C_{D,i}^{k+1} - C_{v,i}^{k+1}; \quad R_i^{k+1} = -C_{D,i}^{k+1} + C_{v,i}^{k+1}; \quad S_i^{k+1} = 1 + 2C_{D,i}^{k+1}$$

$$Q_i^{k+1} = \left(1 - b_i^{1,k+1}\right) n_i^k + \sum_{m=1}^{k-1} \left(b_i^{m,k+1} - b_i^{m+1,k+1}\right) n_i^{k-m} + b_i^{k,k+1} n_i^0. \quad (21)$$

At k, for $k \geq 1$ and $1 \leq i \leq N_x - 1$, Eq. (19) is a set of linear equations for $n(x_i, t_{k+1})$ and can be written as

$$\begin{bmatrix} S_1^{k+1} & R_1^{k+1} & 0 & & \cdots & & 0 \\ P_1^{k+1} & S_2^{k+1} & R_2^{k+1} & & & & \\ 0 & \ddots & \ddots & \ddots & \ddots & & \\ & & P_{i-1}^{k+1} & S_i^{k+1} & R_i^{k+1} & & \\ \vdots & & \ddots & \ddots & \ddots & \ddots & 0 \\ & & & & P_{N_x-3}^{k+1} & S_{N_x-2}^{k+1} & R_{N_x-2}^{k+1} \\ 0 & & \cdots & & 0 & P_{N_x-2}^{k+1} & S_{N_x-1}^{k+1} \end{bmatrix} \begin{bmatrix} n_1^{k+1} \\ n_2^{k+1} \\ \vdots \\ n_i^{k+1} \\ \vdots \\ n_{N_x-2}^{k+1} \\ n_{N_x-1}^{k+1} \end{bmatrix} = \begin{bmatrix} Q_1^{k+1} \\ Q_2^{k+1} \\ \vdots \\ Q_i^{k+1} \\ \vdots \\ Q_{N_x-2}^{k+1} \\ Q_{N_x-1}^{k+1} \end{bmatrix}$$

$$(22)$$

with the boundary conditions as $n(0,t) = n(L,t) = 0$. The charge carrier density $n(x_i, t_k)$ values on the right hand side of the matrix for all the previous time steps are known for all grid points. The matrix in Eq. (22) is a tri-diagonal matrix since the central three diagonal elements on the left hand side of the matrix are nonzero.

The solution $n(x_i, t_{k+1})$ of the VOTFDDE can be obtained by solving the matrix in Eq. (22) using the forward elimination and backward substitution method as outlined below. After forward elimination, coefficient P will become zero, coefficient R is unchanged and the new value of the ith-element of coefficient Q and S is calculated as:

$$S_i^{k+1} \leftarrow S_i^{k+1} - \left(\frac{P_{i-1}^{k+1}}{S_{i-1}^{k+1}}\right) R_{i-1}^{k+1}; \quad 2 \leq i \leq N_x - 1. \quad (23)$$

$$Q_i^{k+1} \leftarrow Q_i^{k+1} - \left(\frac{P_{i-1}^{k+1}}{S_{i-1}^{k+1}}\right) Q_{i-1}^{k+1}; \quad 2 \leq i \leq N_x - 1. \quad (24)$$

The new value for the matrix in Eq. (22) becomes

$$\begin{bmatrix} S_1^{k+1} & R_1^{k+1} & 0 & \cdots & & & 0 \\ 0 & S_2^{k+1} & R_2^{k+1} & & & & \\ & \ddots & \ddots & & & & \vdots \\ & & \ddots & S_i^{k+1} & R_i^{k+1} & \ddots & \\ \vdots & & & \ddots & \ddots & 0 & \\ & & & & S_{N_x-2}^{k+1} & R_{N_x-2}^{k+1} \\ 0 & \cdots & & & 0 & S_{N_x-1}^{k+1} \end{bmatrix} \begin{bmatrix} n_1^{k+1} \\ n_2^{k+1} \\ \vdots \\ n_i^{k+1} \\ \vdots \\ n_{N_x-2}^{k+1} \\ n_{N_x-1}^{k+1} \end{bmatrix} = \begin{bmatrix} Q_1^{k+1} \\ Q_2^{k+1} \\ \vdots \\ Q_i^{k+1} \\ \vdots \\ Q_{N_x-2}^{k+1} \\ Q_{N_x-1}^{k+1} \end{bmatrix}.$$

$$(25)$$

Then, one performs backward substitution to obtain the solution $n(x_i, t_k)$. From Eq. (25), one gets the solution at $n(x_{Nx-1}, t_{k+1})$ as

$$n_{N_x-1}^{k+1} = \frac{Q_{N_x-1}^{k+1}}{S_{N_x-1}^{k+1}}. \tag{26}$$

For i^{th}-element of $n(x_i, t_{k+1})$, it is obtained as

$$n_i^{k+1} = \frac{1}{S_i^{k+1}} \left(Q_i^{k+1} - R_i^{k+1} n_{i+1}^{k+1} \right); \quad 1 \le i \le N_x - 2. \tag{27}$$

3.2. *Numerical scheme for electric potential and electric field*

After obtaining the solution for the charge carrier density, the electric potential is obtained through the Poisson equation. Centered difference scheme is employed to discretize the spatial derivative in Eq. (7). Thus, the approximation of Poisson equation is written as

$$\frac{\partial^2 V(x_i, t_{k+1})}{\partial x^2} = -\frac{qn(x_i, t_{k+1})}{\varepsilon_r \varepsilon_0}. \tag{28}$$

$$\left[\frac{V(x_{i+1}, t_{k+1}) - 2V(x_i, t_{k+1}) + V(x_{i-1}, t_{k+1})}{(\Delta x)^2} \right] = -\frac{en(x_i, t_{k+1})}{\varepsilon_r \varepsilon_0} + O\left((\Delta x)^2 \right). \tag{29}$$

Let's define

$$V(x_i, t_k) = V(i\Delta x, k\Delta t) = V_i^k. \tag{30}$$

Equation (29) can then be rewritten as

$$V_{i-1}^{k+1} - 2V_i^{k+1} + V_{i+1}^{k+1} = -\frac{e(\Delta x)^2}{\varepsilon_r \varepsilon_0} n_i^{k+1}. \tag{31}$$

At k, for $k \ge 1$ and $1 \le i \le N_x - 1$, Eq. (31) is a set of linear equations for $V(x_i, t_{k+1})$ and can be written as

$$
\begin{bmatrix}
-2 & 1 & 0 & & \cdots & & 0 \\
1 & -2 & 1 & & & & \\
0 & \ddots & \ddots & \ddots & \ddots & & \vdots \\
& & 1 & -2 & 1 & & \\
\vdots & & \ddots & \ddots & \ddots & \ddots & 0 \\
& & & 1 & -2 & 1 & \\
0 & & \cdots & & 0 & 1 & -2
\end{bmatrix}
\begin{bmatrix}
V_1^{k+1} \\
V_2^{k+1} \\
\vdots \\
V_i^{k+1} \\
\vdots \\
V_{N_x-2}^{k+1} \\
V_{N_x-1}^{k+1}
\end{bmatrix}
= -\frac{e\,(\Delta x)^2}{\varepsilon_r \varepsilon_0}
\begin{bmatrix}
n_1^{k+1} + \frac{\varepsilon_r \varepsilon_0}{e(\Delta x)^2} V_0^{k+1} \\
n_2^{k+1} \\
\vdots \\
n_i^{k+1} \\
\vdots \\
n_{N_x-2}^{k+1} \\
n_{N_x-1}^{k+1} + \frac{\varepsilon_r \varepsilon_0}{e(\Delta x)^2} V_{N_x}^{k+1}
\end{bmatrix}
$$

$$\text{(32)}$$

where the boundary conditions are $V(0,t) = V_a$ (applied bias) and $V(L,t) = 0$. All the values of the charge density $\rho(x_i, t_{k+1})$ on the right hand side of the matrix are known for all grid points. The matrix in Eq. (32) is a tri-diagonal matrix since the central three diagonal elements on the left hand side of the matrix are nonzero.

By following the similar steps used to obtain the solution for the charge carrier density, based on the forward elimination and backward substitution method, the matrix in Eq. (32) could be solved to obtain the electric potential. After that, the localized electric field at each grid point is solved via the following equation. The centered difference method is used to discretize the electric field. Thus, the approximation of the localized electric field is

$$
E\,(x_i, t_{k+1}) = -\frac{\partial V\,(x_i, t_{k+1})}{\partial x}.
\tag{33}
$$

$$
E\,(x_i, t_{k+1}) = -\left[\frac{V\,((i+1)\,\Delta x,\,(k+1)\,\Delta t) - V\,((i-1)\,\Delta x,\,(k+1)\,\Delta t)}{2\Delta x}\right] + O\,(\Delta x).
\tag{34}
$$

Define

$$
E\,(x_i, t_k) = E\,(i\Delta x, k\Delta t) = E_i^k.
\tag{35}
$$

Equation (33) can then be rewritten as

$$
E_i^{k+1} = -\left[\frac{V_{i+1}^{k+1} - V_{i-1}^{k+1}}{2\Delta x}\right].
\tag{36}
$$

The electric fields at the boundaries are obtained as

$$
E\,(0, t_{k+1}) = E_0^{k+1} = -\left[\frac{V_1^{k+1} - V_0^{k+1}}{\Delta x}\right],
\tag{37}
$$

$$
E\,(L, t_{k+1}) = E_{N_x}^{k+1} = -\left[\frac{V_{N_x}^{k+1} - V_{N_x-1}^{k+1}}{\Delta x}\right].
\tag{38}
$$

3.3. *Numerical scheme for current density*

Centered difference method is used to discretize the space derivative of the total (single carrier type) current density. Thus, the approximation of the total current density at position $x_i = i\Delta x$ is written as

$$J_T(x_i, t_{k+1}) = en(x_i, t_{k+1})\mu E(x_i, t_{k+1}) - eD\frac{\partial n(x_i, t_{k+1})}{\partial x}, \tag{39}$$

$$J_T(x_i, t_{k+1})$$

$$= en(i\Delta x, (k+1)\Delta t)\mu E_x(i\Delta x, (k+1)\Delta t)$$

$$- eD\left[\frac{n((i+1)\Delta x, (k+1)\Delta t) - n((i-1)\Delta x, (k+1)\Delta t)}{2\Delta x}\right] + O(\Delta x). \tag{40}$$

Let's define

$$J_T(x_i, t_k) = J_T(i\Delta x, k\Delta t) = J_{Ti}^k. \tag{41}$$

Equation (40) can be rewritten as

$$J_i^{k+1} = en_i^{k+1}\mu E_i^{k+1} - eD\left[\frac{n_{i+1}^{k+1} - n_{i-1}^{k+1}}{2\Delta x}\right]. \tag{42}$$

The total current density at the boundaries are obtained as

$$J_T(0, t_{k+1}) = J_{T0}^{k+1} = -\left[\frac{n_1^{k+1} - n_0^{k+1}}{\Delta x}\right], \tag{43}$$

$$J_T(L, t_{k+1}) = J_{TNx}^{k+1} = -\left[\frac{n_{N_x}^{k+1} - n_{N_x-1}^{k+1}}{\Delta x}\right]. \tag{44}$$

4. Case Studies of Dispersive Charge Transport

An organic semiconductor thin rod of pentacene ($C_{22}H_{14}$) is considered in the case study. The length of the rod is 0.5 μm and the diameter of the rod is negligibly small compared to the length of the rod. A bias of 5 V is applied at both ends of the rod and the temperature of the rod is kept at 300 K. A square pulse with density of 5000 cm^{-3} charge carriers is injected at one end of the rod ($x = 0$) and they are collected at the opposite end of the rod ($x = L$). The mobility of the charge carriers is 0.02 cm^2/Vs, the diffusion coefficient D is obtained through the Einstein relationship $D = \mu k_B T/e = 5.172 \times 10^{-4}$ cm^{2}s^{-1}. The transport of charge carriers in the rod is represented using an one-dimensional variable order time-fractional drift-diffusion equation (VOTFDDE) since its area is negligible.

The simulation begins with setting up the initial condition and boundary conditions for electric potential, electric field, and charge carrier density. Secondly, the charge carrier density is obtained by solving the VOTFDDE. Thirdly, the electric potential and electric field are obtained by solving the Poisson equation after the information of charge carrier density is obtained. The electric field is then used again to solve for the next time step charge carrier density through the VOTFDDE. These two alternating procedures are repeated till the simulation reaches the maximum simulation time. In each time step, the velocity and total current density of charge carrier are also obtained. Finally, the simulation is stopped. The homogeneity of the material is emulated by setting the fractional derivative order to be a constant value or a function of space. The fractional derivative order values are taken to be $\alpha = 1$ (standard diffusion), $\alpha = 0.50$, $\alpha(x,t) = 1 - x/L$ (crystalline-amorphous-mixed structure) and $\alpha(x,t) = x/L$ for $0 < x < L$ (amorphous-crystalline-mixed structure).

4.1. *Results and discussions*

Fig. 1(a) shows the charge carrier density obtained for standard diffusion ($\alpha = 1$) at different times. It can be seen that the pulse of the charge carrier is maintained as Gaussian-like distribution when the charge carriers are swept across the device having the homogeneous crystalline-like structure. This indicates that the entire pulse of the charge carriers could leave the device at about the same time before the second pulse of charge carriers is injected into the device. This yields the device to have higher frequency response if the transport dynamics of charge carriers follows the normal diffusion process. Fig. 1(b) shows the charge carrier density obtained for $\alpha = 0.50$ at different times. At the beginning, the pulse of the charge carriers deviates slightly from the Gaussian distribution. But, the pulse broadening of the charge carriers due to the sub-diffusive process causes the distribution of charge carrier to follow a long-tail distribution. Hence, charge carriers are distributed throughout the device while moving out from the device.

Fig. 2(a) shows the charge carrier density obtained for $\alpha(x,t) = x/L$ at different times. The fractional derivative order is linearly increasing from zero to one as the charge carriers are moving from where they are injected into the device to the other end of the device where they are being swept out from the device. The increasing of the fractional derivative order is to represent the inhomogeneity of the material where the inhomogeneity is changing from an amorphous-like structure to a crystalline-like structure. This configuration emulates the amorphous-crystalline-mixed structure of pentacene. It can be seen that the square pulse of the charge carriers quickly broadens as they are moving out from the device. This is because charge carriers are injected first into the amorphous-like structure and moving with sub-diffusive transport dynamics. As the charge carriers are moving towards the other end of the device with crystalline-like structure, charge carriers are moving with normal diffusion process and trying to retain a Gaussian-like distribution. Hence, the pulse broadening effect is impeding with time. Fig. 2(b) shows the charge carrier density obtained for $\alpha(x,t) = 1 - x/L$ at different times. The fractional

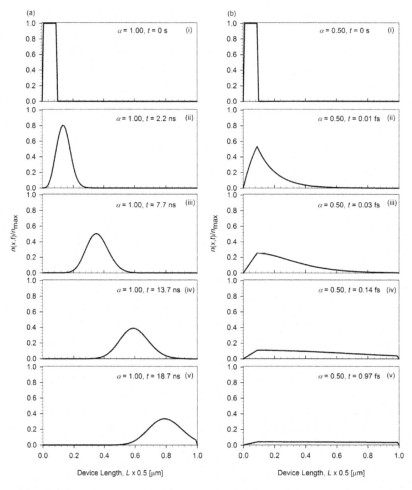

Fig. 1. (a) and (b) represent the charge carrier density obtained for $\alpha = 1$ (standard diffusion) and $\alpha = 0.50$ at different times.

derivative order is linearly decreasing from one approaching to zero as the charge carriers are moving from where they are injected into the device to the other end of the device where they are being swept out from the device. The decreasing of the fractional derivative order is to represent the inhomogeneity of the material where the inhomogeneity is changing from a crystalline-like structure to an amorphous-like structure. This configuration emulates the crystalline-amorphous-mixed structure of pentacene. It can be seen that the pulse maintains a Gaussian-like distribution at a short time before the pulse broadens throughout the whole device. This is because the charge carriers are injected first at the region which represents a crystalline-like structure that causes the charge carriers moving with the normal diffusion process. However, the pulse is getting broader in (square) shape when they are moving towards the other end of the device. This is because the region near the other end

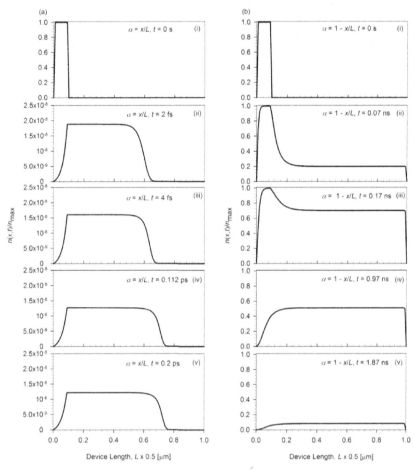

Fig. 2. (a) and (b) represent the charge carrier density obtained for $\alpha(x,t) = x/L$ and $\alpha(x,t) = 1 - x/L$ at different times.

of the device represents an amorphous structure that causes charge carriers moving with sub-diffusive transport dynamics.

Since the profiles of the current density obtained for all the values of the fractional derivative order replicated the corresponding profiles of the charge carrier density, thus the interpretation of the profile of the charge carrier density can be also used to explain the behavior of the current density. Thus, only few examples of the current density profiles are presented in this paper. Fig. 3(a) shows the current density obtained for $\alpha(x,t) = x/L$ at different times. It can be seen that the square pulse of the current density broadens as the current pulse is moving across the device. This is because charge carriers are moving with sub-diffusive transport dynamics within the amorphous-like region of the device. As the current pulse is progressively moving towards the crystalline-like region at the other end of the device, the current pulse is trying to retain a Gaussian-like distribution. Hence, the

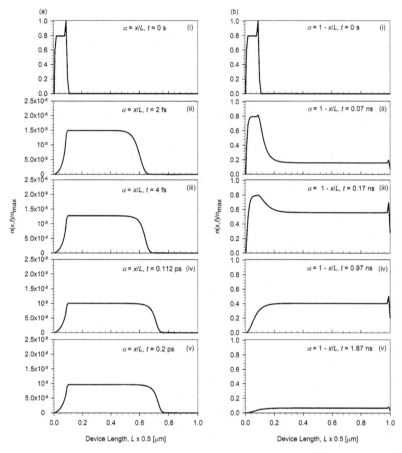

Fig. 3. (a) and (b) represent the current density obtained for $\alpha(x,t) = x/L$ and $\alpha(x,t) = 1 - x/L$ at different times.

pulse broadening effect is decreasing with time. Fig. 3(b) shows the current density obtained for $\alpha(x,t) = 1 - x/L$ at different times. It can be seen that the current pulse maintains a Gaussian-like distribution for a short time before the current pulse begins to broaden when the charge carriers are being swept across the device. This is because the charge carriers are first moving from a crystalline-like structure to an amorphous-like structure that causes the charge carriers moving with the sub-diffusive transport dynamics.

5. Conclusion

The time-fractional drift-diffusion equation is employed to simulate the transport dynamics of charge carriers in pentacene. The types of structures of pentacene emulated in this work are ranging from homogenous crystalline ($\alpha = 1$) structure to homogeneous amorphous ($\alpha \rightarrow 0$) structure and also including the inhomogeneous crystalline-amorphous-mixed ($\alpha(x,t) = 1 - x/L$) structure and amorphous-crystalline-mixed $(\alpha(x,t) = x/L)$ structure. This is done through simulating the transport dynamics of charge carrier using different values or functions of the fractional derivative order. The fractional-time derivative operator and spatial derivative operator of the time-fractional drift-diffusion equation are discretized respectively using the implicit difference scheme and the centered difference scheme. When charge carriers are moving in a homogenous crystalline-like structure, the profile of the injected square pulse changes to a Gaussian-like profile. However, the profile of the injected square pulse broadens significantly when charge carriers are moving in a homogeneous amorphous-like structure. For inhomogeneous amorphous-crystalline-mixed structure, even if the profile of the injected square pulse seems to be initially broader but the pulse broadening effect is impeded as charge carriers are moving towards to the other end of the device with crystalline-like structure. In contrast, the pulse broadening of the injected square pulse is getting serious with time while charge carriers are moving across the device having the inhomogeneous crystalline-amorphous-mixed structure. Therefore, either homogenous crystalline-like structure or inhomogeneous amorphous-crystalline-mixed structure can be used in order to reduce the pulse broadening effect.

Acknowledgments

The authors are extremely grateful to the University of Malaya for PRPUM Grant (CG010-2013) and Ministry of Education for funding support under Long Term Research Grant Scheme (LR003-2011A).

References

1. H. Shirakawa, A. McDiarmid and A. Heeger, *Chem. Commun.*, 1-4 (2003).
2. S. Yoo, B. Domercq and B. Kippelen, *Appl. Phys. Lett.* **85**, 5427 (2004).
3. M. Kitamura, T. Imada and Y. Arakawa, *Appl. Phys. Lett.* **83**, 3410 (2003).
4. M. Kitamura and Y. Arakawa, *J. Phys.: Condens. Matter* **20**, 184011 (2008).
5. H. Scher and E. W. Montroll, *Phys. Rev. B* **12**, 2455 (1975).
6. M. Silver and L. Cohen, *Phys. Rev. B* **15**, 3276 (1977).
7. G. Lanzani, *Photophysics of molecular materials: From single molecules to single crystals* (Wiley-VCH, Weinheim, 2006).
8. R. Metzler, E. Barkai and J. Klafter, *Phys. Rev. Lett.* **82**, 3563 (1999).
9. R. Metzler, *Phys. Rev. E* **63**, 012103 (2001).
10. E. Barkai, *Phys. Rev. E* **63**, 046118 (2001).
11. F. Liu, V. Anh and I. Turner, *J. Comput. Appl. Math.* **166**, 209 (2004).
12. W. R. Scheider and W. Wyss, *J. Math. Phys.* **27**, 2782 (1989).
13. R. T. Sibatov and V. V. Uchaikin, *Phys.-Uspekhi* **52**, 1019 (2009).
14. B. J. West and S. Picozzi, *Phys. Rev. E* **65**, 037106 (2002).
15. S. C. Lim and S. V. Muniandy, *Phys. Rev. E* **66**, 021114 (2002).
16. R. Metzler and J. Klafter, *Phys. Rev. E* **61**, 6308 (2001).
17. A. Compte, *Phys. Rev. E* **53**, 4191 (1996).
18. A. I. Saichev and G. M. Zaslavsky, *Chaos* **7**, 753 (1997).
19. H. C. Fogedby, *Phys. Rev. Lett.* **73**, 2517 (1994).
20. Y. Lin and C. Xu, *J. Comp. Phys.* **225**, 153–1552 (2007).

21. H. Sun, W. Chen, C. Li and Y. Chen, *Int. J. Bifurcat. Chaos* **22**, 1250085 (2012).
22. R. T. Sibatov and V. V. Uchaikin, arXiv:1310.0415v1 [cond-mat.dis-nn] (2013).
23. I. Podlubny, Fractional Differential Equations: *An Introduction to Fractional Derivatives, Fractional Differential Equations, to Methods of Their Solution and Some of Their Applications* (Academic Press, San Diego, 1999).

7th Jagna International Workshop (2014)
International Journal of Modern Physics: Conference Series
Vol. 36 (2015) 1560009 (6 pages)
© The Author
DOI: 10.1142/S2010194515600095

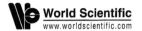

World Scientific
www.worldscientific.com

Bier-Astumian relation, fluctuation theorem and their possible applications

Mark Nolan P. Confesor

*Department of Physics, MSU-Iligan Institute of Technology,
Iligan City, 9200, Philippines*
marknolan2006@gmail.com

Published 2 January 2015

Fluctuations in the spatial position of a probe particle that is driven far from equilibrium can provide valuable information about the driving force. Analysis of the position fluctuation is through the fluctuation theorem (FT) and a generalized detailed balance called Bier-Astumian relation (BA). Here we show the usefulness of the BA for mapping potential landscapes of a particle confined in a potential field. We also demonstrate how the FT can be used to extract the driving force for a particle driven by a constant force.

Keywords: Detailed balance condition; fluctuation theorem.

1. Introduction

There have been great strides in fully developing nanotechnology due to possible uses in medicine, computation and advanced materials among others. Interestingly, such envisioned application of nanotechnology presents fundamental questions in physics such as in the understanding of the effect of thermal noise on the operation of sub-μm sized motors in statistical mechanics [1].

For small systems, the presence of thermal noise naturally leads to fluctuations in some observable quantities conduit to the operation of a particular bio/chem/mechanical operation [2]. One case is when thermal noise leads to the fluctuation in position of a kinesin molecular motor moving in a microtubule [3]. The approach of extracting useful information on the thermodynamics of a system from fluctuating observables has become experimentally practical through the use of μm-sized colloidal beads as probe particles attached to the system of interest, such as beads attached to a F_1-ATPase [4], optically trapped beads dragged in water [5] and an optically trapped bead under a temperature gradient [6,7].

In this article we will present two methods that can be used to analyze the fluctuating position of the probe particle. Our approach is not to provide rigorous mathematical treatment of the methods but rather we will focus more on how such methods can be used to extract thermodynamic variables in the system at hand.

2. Bier-Astumian Relation

For systems in thermodynamic equilibrium, the Detailed Balance (DB) leads to the Boltzmann distribution being the stationary solution of the Master's equation. The DB is basically a measure of reversibility,

$$\frac{P\left(x_a \rightarrow x_b; \Delta t\right)}{P\left(x_b \rightarrow x_a; \Delta t\right)} = \frac{P_{eq}\left(x_b\right)}{P_{eq}\left(x_a\right)} \tag{1}$$

where $P\left(x_i \rightarrow x_j\right)$ is the transition probability to move from position x_i to x_j and $P_{eq}\left(x\right)$ is the position probability distribution [8]. We note that LHS of Eq. 1 is a ratio of two time dependent functions while on the RHS this time dependence vanishes. In Ref. [9], the DB was generalized (the Bier-Astumian relation) to cases when particles are moving in medium with a spatial gradient of a thermodynamic variable $F(x)$, i.e. phoretic transport. For instance in diffusiophoresis particles move due to the presence of solute concentration gradients and in electrophoresis when there is an electric potential gradient [10]. The Bier-Astumian relation (BA) has the form,

$$\frac{P\left(x_a \rightarrow x_b; \Delta t\right)}{P\left(x_b \rightarrow x_a; \Delta t\right)} = e^{-\frac{\Delta G}{k_B T}} \tag{2}$$

where $\Delta G = G\left(F\left(x_b\right)\right) - G\left(F\left(x_a\right)\right)$ and $G\left(F\left(x\right)\right)$ is the free energy. $k_B T$ is the Boltzman factor. In thermophoresis, the free energy difference is updated to include the kinetic energy difference between x_a and x_b [6].

We performed brownian dynamic simulation of a probe particle trapped in a harmonic well to check the validity of the BA, schematics of the set-up is shown in Figure 1.a. The probe particle dynamics is described by the Langevin equation of the form [11],

$$\gamma \frac{dx}{dt} = -kx + \xi(t) \tag{3}$$

where $\gamma = 6\pi\eta a$ (0.017 pN·s/μm), k (1.37 pN/μm) is the trap stiffness and $\xi(t)$ is a white noise with $\langle \xi(t) \rangle = 0$ and $\langle \xi(t)\xi(t') \rangle = 2\gamma k_B T \delta(t - t')$ ($k_B T = 0.004$ pN·μm). Probe position is computed via the time difference form of Eq. 3. Each simulation generated trajectories consisting of 10^4 particle positions in intervals of $\Delta t = 1$ ms. In the inset of Figure 2.a we plot the probe position probability distribution which is well fitted by a normal distribution as expected for a harmonic trap. As a means of checking, the trap stiffness value was recovered from the standard deviation, $\langle \Delta x^2 \rangle$, via the relation, $k = \frac{k_B T}{\langle \Delta x^2 \rangle}$ and from the expected form of the autocorrelation function, $\langle x(t + \Delta t)x(t) \rangle \sim \exp\left[-\frac{t}{\tau}\right]$, where $k = \frac{\gamma}{\tau}$ [11]. In Figure 2.b we plot the

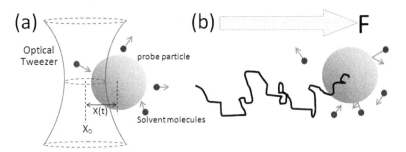

Fig. 1. (a) Probe particle trapped in an optical tweezer. Thermal fluctuations causes the probe particle to deviate from the trap center (X_0). (b) Illustration of a typical trajectory of a probe particle under an external force contains a stochastic and a net drift component.

transition probabilities for the probe particle to jump from $x = 0$ (the trap center) to a position x, $P(0 \to x; \Delta t)$, and the inverse transition probabilities, $P(x \to 0; \Delta t)$. As expected both transition probabilities show different profiles for different time intervals where the profile spread more for $\Delta t = 10$ ms than for $\Delta t = 2$ ms. From the Smoluchowski equation for a particle trapped in a harmonic well, the transition probabilities are computed and take the form [11],

$$P(x \to x'; \Delta t) = F(\Delta t) \exp\left[\frac{k\left[x - x' \exp\left(-\frac{\Delta t}{\tau}\right)\right]^2}{2k_B T \left[1 - \exp\left(-\frac{2\Delta t}{\tau}\right)\right]} \right], \tag{4}$$

where $F(\Delta t)$ is a prefactor. As observed, the spreading of $P(x \to x'; \Delta t)$ increases for bigger Δt. Furthermore, one can then easily show that from the transition probabilities, Eq. 4, the BA holds,

$$\frac{P(x_a \to x_b; \Delta t)}{P(x_b \to x_a; \Delta t)} = \exp\left[\frac{k}{2} \frac{x_a{}^2 - x_b{}^2}{k_B T}\right] = \exp\left[-\frac{\Delta G}{k_B T}\right]. \tag{5}$$

Simulation results also provide validity of the BA as seen by the recovery of the trapping potential well from the ratio of the transition probabilities, $\frac{\Delta U(x)}{k_B T} = \log\left(\frac{P(x \to 0; \Delta t)}{P(0 \to x; \Delta t)}\right)$. The computed potential wells were found to be in excellent agreement with that obtained by the traditional method of inverting the Boltzmann distribution, i.e. $U(x) = -k_B T \log P_{eq}(x)$ as shown in Figure 2.c.

3. Fluctuation Theorem

Generally the fluctuation theorem quantifies the asymmetry in the entropy production of a given system. It is written as,

$$\lim_{\Delta t \to \infty} \frac{k_B}{\Delta t} \ln\left[\frac{P_{\Delta t}(\sigma)}{P_{\Delta t}(-\sigma)}\right] = \sigma \tag{6}$$

where σ is the entropy production and $P_{\Delta t}(\sigma)$ is the time dependent probability distribution for the entropy production [3]. For a colloidal bead immersed in a medium (equilibrated with temperature T) and under an external force, F, the

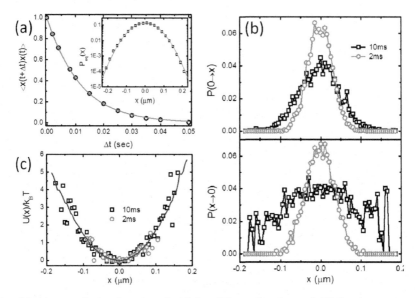

Fig. 2. (a) Autocorrelation function of $x(t)$ for different lag times. Solid line is an exponential fit, $\langle x(t + \Delta t)x(t) \rangle = \exp\left[-\Delta t/\tau\right]$ where $\tau = 0.012s$. Inset shows the probability distribution of the particle position. Fitting curve is a normal distribution fitting with $\langle x \rangle = 0\mu m$ and $\langle \Delta x^2 \rangle = 3 \times 10^{-3}\mu m^2$. (b) Transition probabilities computed for transition from the trap center ($x = 0\mu m$) to a position x and vice versa. (c) Trapping potential as recovered by using the BA (open symbols) and through inverting the Boltzman distribution (solid line).

entropy production is just the rate of heat exchange (Q) of the particle to the bath at some time interval Δt, i.e. $\sigma = Q/T\Delta t$. Furthermore, the heat exchange is given by $Q = \vec{F}\cdot\vec{\Delta x}$ (1-dim), where Δx is the particle incremental step. For the case when $F = 0$ pN, the ratio of $P_{\Delta t}(\sigma)/P_{\Delta t}(-\sigma)$ equals 1 since there is equal probability for the particle to take $+\Delta x$ and $-\Delta x$, i.e. only when there is driving that the ratio is different from 1. In this section we will show the usefulness of the FT in extracting the driving force of a probe particle subjected to a constant external forcing, schematics in Figure 1.b. We performed brownian dynamic simulation of a Langevin equation of the form,

$$\gamma\frac{dx}{dt} = F + \xi(t) \tag{7}$$

where we varied F from 0.0 pN $\rightarrow$ 0.04 pN. The distribution of σ is plotted in the inset of Figure 3.a for two different Δt for the case when $F = 0.01$ pN. We have observed that at longer Δt the asymmetry of the distribution becomes more pronounced. Furthermore, we also verified the validity of the FT for different Δt as shown in Figure 3.a. The practical use of the FT is elucidated in Figure 3.b, where we generate particle trajectories corresponding to different F. We then construct the corresponding probability distribution of Δx for $\Delta t = 0.30$ s and computed the ratio for forward and backward steps as a function of Δx. We see a linear relation between $\ln\left[P_{\Delta t}(\Delta x)/P_{\Delta t}(-\Delta x)\right]$ and Δx such that the y-intercept is the zero point

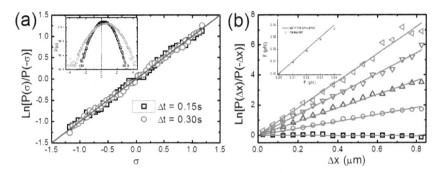

Fig. 3. (a) Verification of the FT, Eq. 6, for the case when $F = 0.01$ pN. Inset shows the distribution of σ for $\Delta t = 0.3$ s and $\Delta t = 0.15$ s (b) Ratio of the forward and backward steps distribution of particle position for different values of F; ($\square$) 0.0 pN, ($\bigcirc$) 0.01 pN, ($\triangle$) 0.02 pN, ($\triangledown$) 0.03 pN and ($\triangleleft$) 0.04 pN . Solid line is a linear fitting with intercept equal to zero. Inset shows the computed force (symbols) to the set values in the simulation (solid line).

as is predicted in Eq. 6. Since $\ln\left[P_{\Delta t}(\Delta x)/P_{\Delta t}(-\Delta x)\right] = \ln\left[P_{\Delta t}(\sigma)/P_{\Delta t}(-\sigma)\right]$ and $\sigma = \frac{F\Delta x}{T\Delta t}$ then the slope of the lines corresponds to $\frac{F}{k_B T}$, i.e. $F = \text{slope}/k_B T$. In the inset of Figure 3.b we plot the computed force from the slope and compared it to the set value of F in the simulation and found good agreements. Lastly, we note that the method described in this section in using FT to measure F was already applied to real systems whose dynamics is described by a Langevin equation similar to Eq. 7, such as the estimation of torque in the rotation of self-propelling dimers [12] and the rotation of F_1-ATPase motor [4].

4. Conclusion

The usefulness of the BA and the FT in extracting thermodynamic variables have been illustrated via simulation for two simple systems. Using the BA the trapping potential was recovered for the case of a probe particle in a harmonic trap. We expect the BA to be able to map even more complicated potential landscapes [13]. Furthermore, the FT was successfully used to recover the driving force for the case of a probe particle under the action of a constant force. The applicability of FT will allow it to measure non-equilibrium driving forces for instance thermophoretic force in thermophoresis [7]. The FT was also used to extract the torque that causes an asymmetric wheel to rotate in the presence of self-propelling particles in the granular scale [14].

Acknowledgments

Insightful discussions with Prof. C. K. Chan and Prof. Pik-Yin Lai are greatly acknowledged.

References

1. R. Phillips and S. R. Quake, *Phys. Today* **59(5)**, 38 (2006).
2. R. Dean Astumian, *Science* **276**, 917 (1997).
3. C. Bustamante et. al, *Phys. Today* **58(7)**, 43 (2005).
4. K. Hayashi et. al, *Phys. Rev. Lett.* **104**, 218103 (2010).
5. D. Andrieux et. al, *Phys. Rev. Lett.* **98**, 150601 (2007).
6. M. N. Confesor and P. Y. Lai, *Chin. J. Phys.* **51**, 522 (2013).
7. M. N. Confesor, P. Y. Lai and C. K. Chan *in preparation.*
8. F. Ritort, *Adv. Chem. Phys.* **137**, (2008).
9. R. Dean Astumian and R. Brody, *J. Phys. Chem. B* **113**, 11459 (2009).
10. J. L. Anderson, *Ann. Rev. of Fluid Mech.* **21**, 61-69 (1989).
11. M. Doi and S. F. Edwards, *The Theory of Polymer Dynamics*, (Clarendon Press, 1998).
12. R. Suzuki, H. R. Jiang and M. Sano, *arXiv:1104.5607.*
13. X. G. Ma, P. Y. Lai and P. Tong, *Soft Matter* **9**, 8826 (2013).
14. E. Hamoy and M. N. Confesor, *to be submitted.*

7th Jagna International Workshop (2014)
International Journal of Modern Physics: Conference Series
Vol. 36 (2015) 1560010 (5 pages)
© The Authors
DOI: 10.1142/S2010194515600101

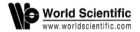
World Scientific
www.worldscientific.com

Robust method of trapping self-propelling particles

Roger Joseph L. Lacubtan

College of Arts and Sciences, Central Mindanao University,
Musuan, 8710, Philippines

Mark Nolan P. Confesor

Department of Physics, MSU-Iligan Institute of Technology,
Iligan City, 9200, Philippines
marknolan2006@gmail.com

Published 2 January 2015

The ability to collect self-propelling particles (SPP) is an essential requirement for possible use of SPP in technological applications. In this paper we proposed a novel way of trapping SPP's, through guided trapping of SPP's in V-shaped trap. We performed brownian dynamic simulation via a modified Escape and Predation model developed by L. Angelani (Phys. Rev. Lett., 2012) to assess the validity of the proposed trapping method.

Keywords: Collecting self-propelling particles; escape and predation.

1. Introduction

Self-propelling particles (SPP) are ubiquitous in nature. SPPs are observed at different length scales; ranging from μm sized motile bacteria to m sized fishes such as whales. Due to huge promising application in medicine, nano-technology, and intelligent controls, there is a myriad of artificial SPP's that have been conceived and experimentally made [1].

In most conceived cases of using μm-sized SPPs in biotechnology, techniques enabling the collection of SPPs are essential. Existing and suggested approaches are the use of funnel shaped gates that leads to the sorting of rod-shaped SPPs to passive ones [2]; use of wedge like obstacles to collect for also rod-like shaped SPPs [3]; and an array of L-shaped obstacles for SPPs moving in circular trajectories [4]. A general mechanism to trap SPPs independent of the shape or the propelling mechanism therefore, has yet to be found.

In this study we propose a novel way of trapping SPPs independent of their shape or the nature of the propulsion with shepherding as our inspiration. In our trapping method we make use of another SPP (chaser) to guide our SPP of interest (target) towards a V-shaped trap for collection same as shepherds do to the sheep.

2. Brownian dynamics simulation

We performed brownian dynamic simulation of an escape and predation model proposed by L. Angelani [5] but with a modification that the targets are not annihilated and that there is a presence of a V-shaped trap. Furthermore, chasers are not allowed to get inside the space enclosed by the V-shaped trap and such space is accessible only to targets.

In the simulation employed, both the chaser and the target has a constant speed set at v_0. However, the direction of motion of either the chaser or target can change due to localized interaction. Specifically the velocity of a particle i (target or chaser) is given by [5],

$$v_i^{(int)} = \alpha v_i^{(al)} + \beta f_i^{(rep)} + \gamma g_i^{(rep)} + \delta f_i^{(al)}. \tag{1}$$

The first term corresponds to the alignment of the particles based on the Vicsek model; particle i next position is on the same direction as the average velocity of the neighboring particles (of the same type) within some radius of the particle i [6]. The second and third term in Equation 1, corresponds to the exclusive volume interaction that causes no particle (chaser or target) to be on the same location. The last term corresponds to the chase or escape force such that a chaser will move towards the direction of a target as the target moves away from the chaser. After the calculation of the velocity of each particle, the next position of the particle is updated by $v_i^{(inst)} \Delta t$, where Δt is the time step. Parameter values used in the simulations are similar to those used in Ref. [5].

3. Escape and predation without annihilation

To better understand the guided trapping mechanism, first we need to assess the chase statistics for the case when there is no V-shaped trap. In the simulation, we incorporate a repulsive boundary condition and varied the concentration ratio of target and chaser from $0.1 \leq \phi \leq 6$ (ϕ = total number of target/total number of chaser). Screenshot images of the simulation are shown in Figure 1.a-c for three concentration regimes of ϕ. Initially the particles are distributed randomly in the simulation box. However, as the simulation progress we observe clustering of same particle species. We note that due to the Vicsek alignment, both the target and chaser exhibit collective motion by themselves. Furthermore, due to the chase and escape force the chasers tend to move towards targets and thus the system exhibits complex collective motion, i.e. collective motion of both the target and chasers is coupled. To quantize the observed collective motion we employ the order parameter,

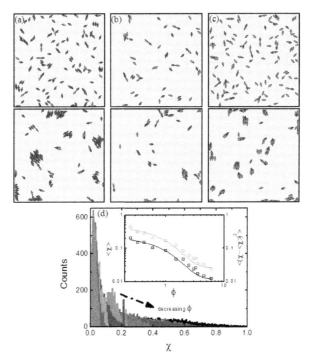

Fig. 1. (Color online) (a-c) Screenshots of the simulation for different concentration ratio ϕ; (a) $\phi < 1$, (b) $\phi = 1$, and (c) $\phi > 1$. The blue particles correspond to the targets while the red particles correspond to the chasers. The upper images correspond to the initial distribution of the particles while the lower images correspond to the steady state (after 1500 simulation runs). (d) Histogram of χ_{chaser} for various ϕ. Inset. The mean and standard deviation of the $P(\chi_{chaser})$ is plotted versus ϕ. Solid line is an exponential decay fit.

χ, given by, $\chi = \frac{1}{N v_0} \left| \sum_j \vec{v}_j \right|$, where N is the total number of targets or chasers and $\vec{v}_j$ is the individual velocity of either a target or a chaser. Particles are all aligned when $\chi = 1$ and there are no particle orientational correlation for $\chi = 0$. In Figure 1.d we plot the distribution of χ_{chaser} for different ϕ. From the distribution of χ_{chaser}, statistical measures such as the mean order parameter, $\langle \chi \rangle$, and the standard deviation $\langle (\chi - \langle \chi \rangle)^2 \rangle$ were extracted. Both the $\langle \chi \rangle$ and $\langle (\chi - \langle \chi \rangle)^2 \rangle$ were found to be exponentially decaying function of ϕ.

Our result may have some biological implications, for instance we observe that at higher concentration of targets, chasers chase mostly by themselves and not in herds as seen by the decrease of χ_{chaser}. However for the case of lower concentration of targets, chasers chase mostly in groups. This behavior of food search is similar to that used by Dictyostelium at environments of low food concentration [7].

4. Guided trapping of target SPPs

The interaction between the SPP (target or chaser) and the V-shaped trap is such that only the SPP velocity component parallel to the trap contributes. Figure 2.a-g

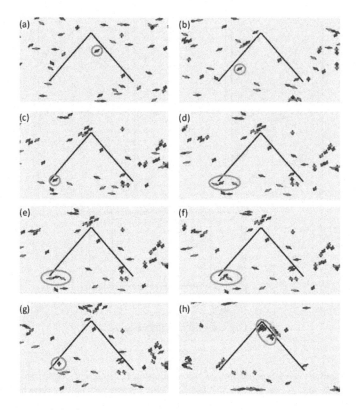

Fig. 2. (Color online) (a-g) Sequential screenshot images of the guided trapping of a target to a V-shaped trap for $\phi = 1$. (h) Trapping at long time.

are simulation screenshots showing one mechanism of a guided trapping of a target SPP to a V-shaped trap for $\phi = 1$. In Figure 2.a-c, the target which initially is located inside the trap has its direction of motion going outside the trap. We note that since there is no other target SPP's near it (no Vicsek interaction) and since no chaser is allowed inside the trap, our target of interest moves in a straight line until it encounters a chaser that causes it to move in the opposite direction. Finally in Figure 2.e-f we see the joint effect of two chasers that cause the target to return inside the trap. We observed that at long time, more target SPP's are trapped inside the trap although their trapping mechanism could be different from the one detailed above. Factors affecting the efficiency of the trapping mechanism such as noise, apex angle of the trap as well as the concentration ratio will be discussed in detail in a separate article [8].

5. Conclusion

The guided trapping of target SPP to a V-shaped trap is possible as verified via Brownian dynamic simulation. This trapping mechanism is robust as it can work on target SPPs of varying shapes and propulsion mechanism since these parameters were not specified in the simulation.

References

1. S. J. Ebbens and J. R. Howse, In pursuit of propulsion at the nanoscale, *Soft Matter* **6**, 726 (2010).
2. P. Galajda, J. Keymer, P. Chaikin, and R. Austin, A wall of funnels concentrates swimming bacteria, *J. Bacteriol.* **189**, 8704 (2007).
3. A. Kaiser, H. Wensik, and H. Löwen, How to Capture Active Particles, *Phys. Rev. Lett.* **108**, 268307 (2012).
4. C. Reichhardt and C. J. Oslon Reichhardt, Active Matter Ratchets with an External Drift, *arXiv:1307.0755v1*
5. L. Angelani, Collective Predation and Escape Strategies, *Phys. Rev. Lett.* **109**, 118104 (2012).
6. T. Vicsek, A. Czirok, E. Ben-Jacob, I. Cohen, and C. Shochet, Novel Type of Phase Transition in a System of Self-Driven Particles, *Phys. Rev. Lett.* **75**, 1226 (1995).
7. B. A. Lazazzera, Quorum sensing and starvation: signals for entry into stationary phase, *Current Opinion in Microbiology* **3**, 177 (2000).
8. R. Lacubtan and M. N. Confesor, in preparation.

7th Jagna International Workshop (2014)
International Journal of Modern Physics: Conference Series
Vol. 36 (2015) 1560011 (11 pages)
© The Authors
DOI: 10.1142/S2010194515600113

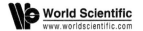

World Scientific
www.worldscientific.com

Mechanism-based model of a mass rapid transit system: A perspective

Erika Fille Legara, Lee Kee Khoon, Hung Gih Guang and Christopher Monterola

*Complex Systems Group, Institute of High Performance Computing, Computing Science,
Agency for Science Technology and Research, 1 Fusionopolis Way, Connexis (North Tower)
Singapore 138632*

Published 2 January 2015

In this paper, we discuss our findings on the spatiotemporal dynamics within the mass rapid transit (MRT) system of Singapore. We show that the trip distribution of Origin-Destination (OD) station pairs follows a power-law, implying the existence of critical OD pairs. We then present and discuss the empirically validated agent-based model (ABM) we have developed. The model allows recreation of the observed statistics and the setting up of various scenarios and their effects on the system, such as increasing the commuter population and the propagation of travel delays within the transportation network. The proposed model further enables identification of bottlenecks that can cause the MRT to break down, and consequently provide foresight on how such disruptions can possibly be managed. This can potentially provide a versatile approach for transport planners and government regulators to make quantifiable policies that optimally balance cost and convenience as a function of the number of the commuting public.

Keywords: Agent-based modelling; transport dynamics; power law; rail transport system.

1. Introduction

A transportation system is a complex system that exhibits collective phenomena resulting from the interaction of its components. The efficiency of transportation networks is crucial in connecting communities as they allow individuals to perform various economic activities– from going to work or school, to shopping and/or making leisure visits. Consequently, there are many intertwined urban issues that surround these systems– from the infrastructures themselves to the passengers/commuters utilizing them. Here, we look into the mass rapid transit system (MRT), which is becoming the foremost public mode of travel worldwide, especially in highly-urbanized cities. It is an economically viable choice since, as the name implies, it caters to larger volumes of public commuters and sends them to their destinations at higher velocities at a given time.

As more and more individuals depend on the MRT, it is important to have a way to objectively assess its reliability and resilience to a growing city and thus, to a growing population. Questions such as the MRT's robustness to breakdowns or if there are "tipping points" present in the system are critical information to policymakers, urban planners, and other stakeholders. To understand these issues, it is necessary to not only look at the MRT infrastructure singly nor just the individual commuters that utilize the system, but more importantly, to also study the interactions of the entities present in the system.

Fortunately, large socio-technical datasets are becoming increasingly available; for public transportation systems, for example, smart fare cards or ticketing data have allowed researchers to gain deeper insights on the travel patterns of commuters. Generally, knowing the prevailing travel demand and the collective behavior of commuters is the first step to a more systematic understanding of such complex system.

In this article, we first report on key statistical features with regard to travel demand of different origin-destination (OD) pairs in Singapore's MRT stations and show that journeys utilizing these pairs exhibit a power-law distribution with an exponent of -1, i.e. there exist a small number of stations that critically serve a large number of commuters. We then discuss a procedure of capturing various MRT dynamics using an agent based model that was first described in reference [1]. Essentially, from the statistical features of the MRT, specifically the arrival times of commuters in stations, we have set up an agent-based model that can infer the travel time distributions for specific OD pairs. The simulation framework has been validated by comparing the results with actual recorded durations of travel from the existing ticketing data. The developed model is then used to explore the spatiotemporal correlation of commuters' travel times with various hypothetical scenarios involving inflation of population at various MRT stations.

2. Collective Phenomena in the Dynamics within the MRT

We discuss below some of the statistics collected and observed from Singapore's contactless smart ticketing card[a] that automatically collects fares for its MRT and bus system. A smart fare card essentially stores spatiotemporal information on a system's commuting public (where the identity of the card holder has been anonymized and the transaction data do not contain any personal information). The MRT of Singapore is estimated to serve around 20% of its total population per day. The smart fare card data in this report cover a duration of one week and contain information on around 14 million journeys that involve the MRT.

2.1. *Travel demand at different times of the day*

Figure 1 shows the typical pattern of ridership in Singapore's MRT. During weekdays, it is characterized by a peak in the morning from 7:30 to 9:30 and another

---

[a]The ticketing dataset was provided by the Singapore Land Transport Authority (LTA).

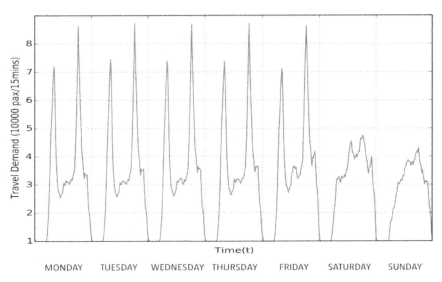

Fig. 1. One week travel demand of commuters in Singapore. The dataset includes more than 14 million journeys within one (1) week across 121 stations.

peak in the evening from 17:30 to 19:30. The distribution is generally more dispersed or uniform across different times during weekends. Note that the wider distribution of commuters' timings in the mornings when they are on their way to work places makes the morning peaks lower than the peaks of the evening rides. The consistency of the distribution within the weekdays point to the existence of a routinary pattern of the commuters; and, this signature is expected to be observed in other existing transport systems as well.

2.2. *Power-law scaling of Origin-Destination pairs*

Power-law scaling is a manifestation of long range correlation and is the most utilized signature in defining a complex system or probing the degree of coupling among agents. A power law temporal distribution of inter-event times implies the existence of memory or the presence of historical dependence of the state of evolving agents; while a power law in space, or loosely, the fractality of spatial patterns, implies the presence of a global interaction of the systems' components. Figure 2 shows that OD distribution exhibits power-law characteristics, i.e. there are very few OD pairs that are heavily utilized by the commuters. For instance, a mere 1% of these critical ODs already account for about 17% of the total journeys. The implication of this result is straightforward– any disruption that will include the most utilized stations will result in a catastrophic failure. In the succeeding sections, we discuss an empirical model presented in Ref. 1 that looks at the possible growth dynamics of MRT stations and how such evolution can impact travel time delays of the global (cumulative) and local (selective) OD pairs.

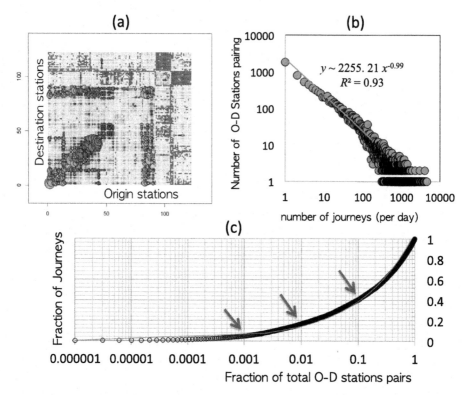

Fig. 2. (Color online) Power-law scaling in Singapore's MRT: (a) Origin-Destination pairs where the size of the circle corresponds to the number of journeys utilizing that pair, while the various colors correspond to the different lines in the system, (b) Log-log plot of the number of OD pairs and the number of commuter journeys it serves showing a power-law with an exponent of -1. A similar result is obtained using Clauset's algorithm in fitting a power law, (c) Semi-log plot of the percentage of commuter journeys and the percent OD pairs utilized. The existence of a power-law distributed utilization of OD pairs indicates that only 0.1% of ODs serve 5% of commuters' journeys, or merely 1% and 10% accounts for 17% and 40% of the journey counts.

2.3. Burst in the in-flow of passengers

Figure 3 shows superimposed plots of the different distributions of inter-tap-in (or inter-arrival) times for select origin stations. We note that the inter-arrival times between two successive commuter agents tapping in at the same origin station exhibits similar statistics across stations and is characterized by "bursts" in the in-flow of passengers (peak hours) separated by prolonged sporadicity in tap-in times (off-peak times). This is manifested by the fat tail of the distribution. This observed statistics is a useful input to the model that will be discussed in the next section.

3. Agent-Based Model

An agent-based model (ABM) is used to capture and reconstruct the observed statistics and emergent phenomena discussed in the previous section. In the model

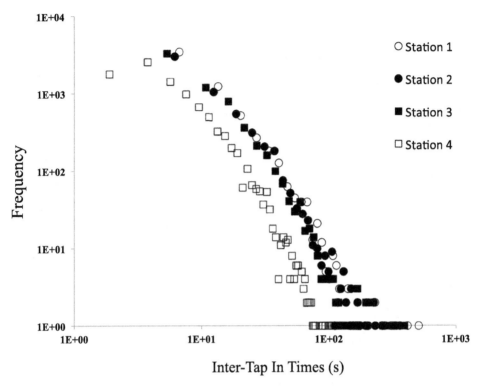

Fig. 3.   Inter-Arrival Time Statistics. Shown are the different inter-arrival time (tap-in) distributions for each origin station under consideration. The distributions are well approximated by a power-law with exponent of 2.4 (average $R^2 \sim 0.91$).

proposed, three (3) types of tractable agent objects are defined: passenger, train, and station.

A schematic diagram of the MRT is shown in Figure 4. In the figure, a track patch/box represents one unit of distance; the system is set up in a manner that it is reminiscent of the actual inter-station distances in the Singapore MRT.

This work is focused on a single uni-directional train track involving trains across a single line in the MRT network system, with the agent object **train** having the following attributes: time of dispatch, velocity, total capacity, current load, and consequently, available capacity. We would like to point interested readers to Ref. 1 for more details on the construction of the ABM.

Results of the model have been validated using empirical tap-out time and duration of travel time statistics. Figure 5 shows selected OD pairs to demonstrate that the travel time distributions obtained in the ABM are in strong agreement with those observed from actual data. Results have been statistically validated as well using Linfoot's criteria: fidelity F, structural content SC, and correlation quantity Q,[2,3] with values $\overline{F} = 0.91$, $\overline{SC} = 0.94$, $\overline{Q} = 0.96$, suggesting that the simulation strongly agrees with the patterns found in the empirical data.

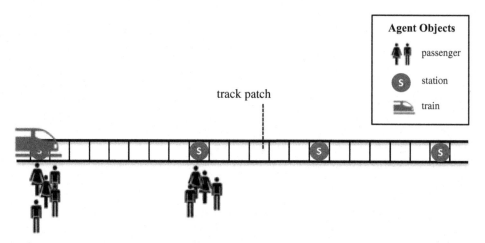

Fig. 4.   Agent Objects in the Railway System Model. The MRT stations are represented by the dark red solid circles marked by numbers. The inter-station distances reflect actual distances. In the model, a unit of distance is defined by a track patch. The approximate dispatch time interval statistics for trains for peak and off-peak are respectively given by: $\mu_{\text{peak}} = 180$, $\sigma_{\text{peak}} = 90$, $\mu_{\text{off-peak}} = 360$, and $\sigma_{\text{off-peak}} = 180$. Time unit is in seconds and the values are guided by actual MRT train dispatch times.

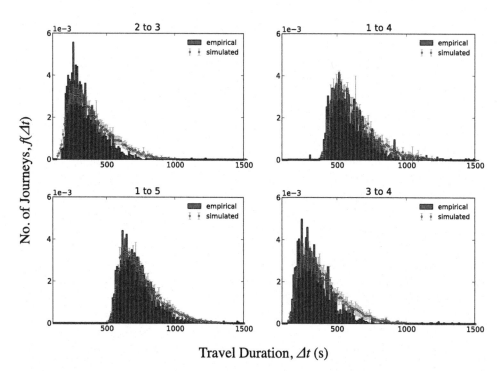

Fig. 5.   (Color online) Total travel time distribution of the ABM model and actual data for various representative OD journeys.

4. Phenomenological Scenarios: Overloading and Overcrowding

Using the validated model, we then explore two phenomenological scenarios: (1) train overloading as a function of the trains' loading capacity and (2) platform overcrowding due to increases in the number of the commuting population. These issues are very *real* in advanced cities where governments are strongly encouraging more citizens to use public transport to unclog busy roads and lessen pollution coming from private vehicles.

For the first case, we have reported that there is a critical train loading capacity C' or a "tipping point" where the durations of travel delays in commuter journeys begin to increase exponentially as the loading capacity decreases to C'. This cascade of delays is very much reminiscent of the sandpile model wherein even the addition of just a single grain of sand can cause an avalanche in the system;[4] similarly, "a small addition in the number of commuters who cannot board the trains can already cause an avalanche of delays" in the system.[1]

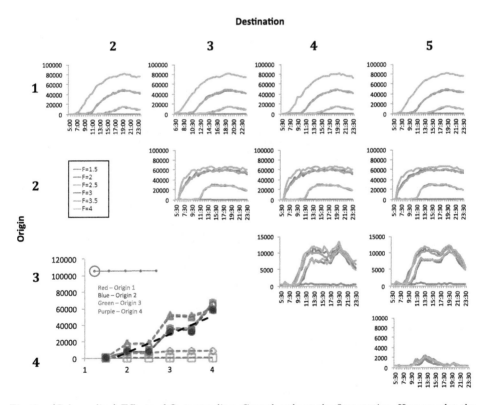

Fig. 6. (Color online) Effects of Overcrowding: Growth only at the first station. Here we plot the temporal behavior of the average travel time delay of commuters along an OD pair, i.e. individuals are grouped together based on the OD pair journey they take. The subgraphs are arranged in a matrix where the rows represent the station origins and the columns represent the destination stations. Shown are the characteristic delay curves resulting from different inflation factor F.

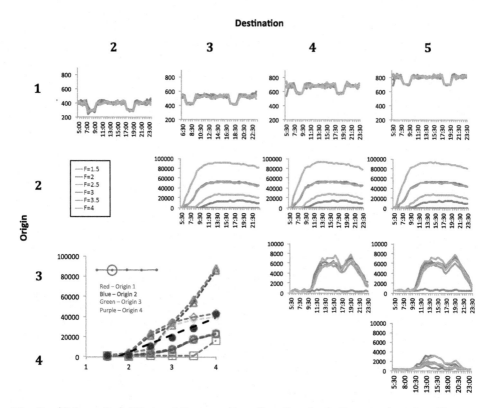

Fig. 7. (Color online) Effects of Overcrowding: Growth only at the second station. Here we plot the temporal behavior of the average travel time delay of commuters along an OD pair, i.e. individuals are grouped together based on the OD pair journey they take. The subgraphs are arranged in a matrix where the rows represent the station origins and the columns represent the destination stations. Shown are the characteristic delay curves resulting from different inflation factor F.

In the second scenario, the effect of the increase in the commuter population on the system is investigated. Simulation results point to some intuitive and counter-intuitive observations. For one, results show that as the population at a particular station is increased by a factor F, the average duration of travel delay linearly increases across the system as well. This result is expected. However, when we zoomed in on specific origin-destination pairs, observations have started to vary. In Figures 6-9, we dissected each of the cases by looking at the average travel time delay of commuters in each OD pair, given the factor of increase F in the total population (distinguished by the colored lines), across the time of day per 30-minute interval. Our aim is to track the dynamics across time especially during peak and off-peak hours when both train and passenger dynamics are significantly altered. The subfigures are arranged such that the rows correspond to the station origin (Stations 1 to 4 denoted by $S_1, ..., S_4$), while the columns correspond to the destination stations S_2 to S_5.

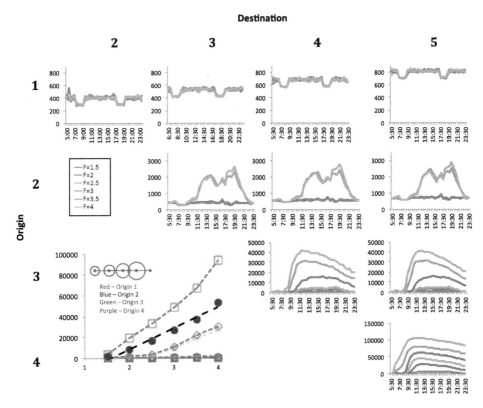

Fig. 8. (Color online) Effects of Overcrowding: Geometrically increasing case. Here we plot the temporal behavior of the average travel time delay of commuters along an OD pair, i.e. individuals are grouped together based on the OD pair journey they take. The subgraphs are arranged in a matrix where the rows represent the station origins and the columns represent the destination stations. Shown are the characteristic delay curves resulting from different inflation factor F.

In Figure 6, a population growth was employed in only one station S_1. The subplots suggest that across the day, all travels coming from origin stations S_1 and S_2 are the most affected (compared to trips coming from S_3 and S_4). Moreover, while journeys originating from S_1 hint to four gradual transitions, the travel delays as functions of F becomes more homogeneous far from S_1. That is, three transitions are observed for journeys originating from S_2, two transitions for S_3 origin ($F = 1.5$ vs all the other Fs), and the system collapses to a single distribution curve for travels originating at S_4. The cascade of delays has an effect on reaching the saturated state and thus homogenizing the system's response as it goes farther from the inflated source. This systematic decrease in the number of transitions is consistently observed in all other cases (Figures 7–9). For instance in Fig. 7, the number of transitions are highest in journeys originating from S_2 where all the passengers are injected. In Figs. 8 and 9, where there is a geometric variation in growth, the number of transitions are highest either in the last two or the first two

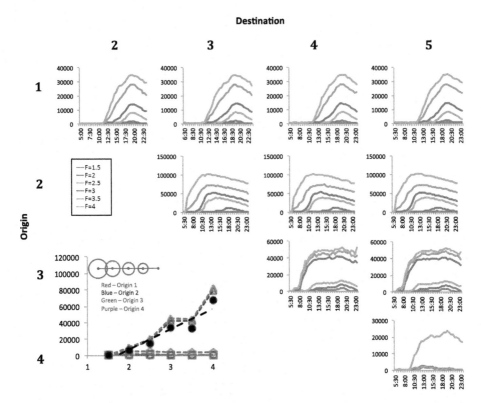

Fig. 9. (Color online) Effects of Overcrowding: Geometrically decreasing case. Here we plot the temporal behavior of the average travel time delay of commuters along an OD pair, i.e. individuals are grouped together based on the OD pair journey they take. The subgraphs are arranged in a matrix where the rows represent the station origins and the columns represent the destination stations. Shown are the characteristic delay curves resulting from different inflation factor F.

origins dependending on whether the commuters are augmented most in the first or the last station, respectively.

The top rows of Figs. 7 and 8 are typical representations of the travel time when there is no overcrowding or addition of agents, where the dips during peak hours is a result of the increase in frequency of train dispatch during this time. Another set of travel delay dips (row 3 in Figs. 6 and 9; row 2 in Fig. 8) are seen during off-peak hours that balances the low frequency of train dispatch by the lower number of commuting passengers. Note that in general, the added passengers in station S_i will have the highest impact on passengers originating from S_{i+1} since at stations farther from $i+1$, portion of the agents that clogged the system will already alight allowing additional capacity in later stations.

5. Conclusion

In this work, we discussed the various statistical features associated with Singapore's MRT system, and described how these empirical observations can be used in developing an agent-based model. We have calibrated and validated our model using the known travel time distribution of commuters. The platform was then used to investigate the impact of inflating the flow volume of commuters in station platforms. Extending the results to phenomenological overcrowding scenarios, we discuss the transient spatiotemporal travel time dynamics and how such result hints to potentially identifying system bottlenecks within a segment of the MRT. Finally, we demonstrate that the durations of travel delays in specific OD pairs, as a result of inflated population, are strongly dependent on how the new commuters are distributed across the train stations. The empirical model reported here is flexible and customizable enough to potentially provide a versatile approach for transport planners and government regulators to make quantifiable policies that optimally balance cost and convenience as a function of the number of the commuting public.

As of this writing, we have also already developed a full-scale agent-based model that concurrently looks at all stations in Singapore. We refer our readers to our recent work appearing in Ref. 5.

Notes and Acknowledgment

We would like to acknowledge LTA Singapore for providing the ticketing data. This research is supported by A*STAR SERC Complex Systems Programme's research grant (1224504056).

References

1. E. F. Legara, C. Monterola, G. Lee, T. Hung, "Critical capacity, travel time delays and travel time distribution of rapid mass transit systems," *Physica A* **406**, pp. 100-106, 2014.
2. F. Huck, C. Fales, N. Halyo, R. Samms, and K. Stacy, "Image gathering and processing: information and fidelity," *J. Opt. Soc. Am. A* **2**, No. 10, 1985.
3. I. Crisologo, R. Batac, A. Longjas, E.F. Legara and C. Monterola, "Visual and auditory cues significantly reduce human's intrinsic biases when tasked to generate a random number sequence," *Intl J of Mod Phys C* **21**, Issue: 5, pp. 567-581, 2010.
4. P. Bak, *How Nature Works: The Science of Self-Organised Criticality*, New York, NY: Copernicus Press, 1996.
5. N. Othman, E. F. Legara, V. Selvam and C. Monterola, "Simulating Congestion Dynamics of Train Rapid Transit using Smart Card Data", *Procedia Computer Science*, Proceedings of the International Conference on Computational Science 2014. DOI: 10.1016/j.procs.2014.05.147

7th Jagna International Workshop (2014)
International Journal of Modern Physics: Conference Series
Vol. 36 (2015) 1560012 (9 pages)
© The Authors
DOI: 10.1142/S2010194515600125

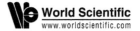
World Scientific
www.worldscientific.com

Critical slowing down in a dynamic duopoly

M. G. O. Escobido

W. Sycip Graduate School of Business, Asian Institute of Management,
123 Paseo de Roxas, Makati City, 1229, Philippines
mescobido@aim.edu
www.aim.edu

N. Hatano

Institute of Industrial Science, University of Tokyo,
Komaba 4-6-1, Meguro, Tokyo 153-8505, Japan
hatano@iis.u-tokyo.ac.jp

Published 2 January 2015

Anticipating critical transitions is very important in economic systems as it can mean survival or demise of firms under stressful competition. As such identifying indicators that can provide early warning to these transitions are very crucial. In other complex systems, critical slowing down has been shown to anticipate critical transitions. In this paper, we investigate the applicability of the concept in the heterogeneous quantity competition between two firms. We develop a dynamic model where the duopoly can adjust their production in a logistic process. We show that the resulting dynamics is formally equivalent to a competitive Lotka-Volterra system. We investigate the behavior of the dominant eigenvalues and identify conditions that critical slowing down can provide early warning to the critical transitions in the dynamic duopoly.

Keywords: Critical slowing down; Lotka-Volterra; complex systems.

1. Introduction

There has been active research to identify signals that can provide early warning prior to critical transitions across different systems.[1,2] Prominent among them is the observation that as the system approaches a critical point, it becomes increasingly slow in recovering from small perturbations. Mathematically, this means that the characteristic return time will increase when one approaches the critical point.[3] This phenomenon has been shown to occur across varied fields such as semiconductor lasers,[4] engineered systems[5] and financial markets.[6] The intent of the paper is to add industrial firms among systems where critical slowing down may anticipate transitions.

Anticipating critical transitions is of fundamental interest in economic systems. For this complex system, changes are not necessarily smooth but can be abrupt, and may cause a critical transition from one dynamical state to another. For instance, the market crash in 1929 brought with it two thousand investment firms and resulted in a structural change in the American banking industry.[7] The more recent financial crisis pushed the global economy into a great recession for which many nations are still reeling from.[8]

Analyzing critical transitions is a strategic concern among firms as it relates to their success or downfall. Yet the analysis can become difficult as the network of firms increase, with each one having a different set of interactions and strategies. Our approach would be to consider the simplest system and investigate its critical transitions. With only two firms competing, duopoly is the simplest form of oligopoly.[9] Even so, it allows for complex interactions depending on the context of the competition and the set-up of the firms[10,11] As such, different forms have been intensively studied to gain insight into the dynamics of industrial organizations.[12]

In this paper, we consider a heterogeneous quantity competition of firms each adjusting their production in a logistic process. We show that the resulting dynamics is governed by Lotka-Volterra equations. We extract the critical points and investigate the dominant eigenvalues around these points. We then identify conditions that critical slowing down can provide early warning prior to critical transitions in the dynamic duopoly.

2. Competition Model

Consider two firms 1 and 2 each with a product competing for the same market. The value of their respective product, as given by its price, depend on the quantities (q_1, q_2) in the market, i.e. $p_i(q_1, q_2), i = 1, 2$. Expanding up to first order one obtains:

$$p_i(q_1, q_2) = p_i(0, 0) + q_1 \frac{\partial p_i}{\partial q_1} + q_2 \frac{\partial p_i}{\partial q_2}. \tag{1}$$

Substituting $\alpha_i = p_i(0, 0)$ and assuming the price decreases with quantity such that $\partial p_i / \partial q_i = -\beta_i$ and $\partial p_i / \partial q_j = -\gamma_{ij}, i \neq j = 1, 2$ we have:

$$p_i(q_1, q_2) = \alpha_i - \beta_i q_i - \gamma_{ij} q_j. \tag{2}$$

One can associate α as the quality of the product in the sense that the higher it is, the greater the product is valued. Rewriting $\beta_i = (\partial q_i / \partial p_i)^{-1}$, the parameter is inversely related to the elasticity concept in economics where one is concerned with the change in the quantities given the change in the price.[13] On the other hand $\gamma_{ij} = (\partial q_j / \partial p_i)^{-1}$ captures how different the products are from each other.[14] For instance, if $\gamma_{ij} > 0$, the product j adversely affects the value of product i and as such can be considered a substitute to product i. For $\gamma_{ij} < 0$, product j increases the value of product i and hence a complement to it; $\gamma_{ij} = 0$ means that product j has no impact on the value of product i.

With the market condition above, we now look at the profit of firm i. The profit $\pi_i(q_i)$ in producing and selling q_i units would be the difference between its revenue and production cost. Its revenue in selling q_i units of the product at price p_i is $p_i q_i$. For zero fixed cost and constant marginal cost m_i, the total cost in production is $m_i q_i$. As such the profit would be given by:

$$\pi_i(q_i) = (\alpha_i - m_i - \beta_i - \gamma_{ij} q_j) q_i. \tag{3}$$

For the firm to maximize its profit, it needs to find the quantity q_i^B that would maximize (3). Taking $\partial \pi_i / \partial q_i$ and equating it to zero and following Cournot's conjecture that the other firm keeps its quantity constant $(\partial q_j / \partial q_i = 0)$ (Cournot, 1960), we obtain the best response of firm i given the output of firm j:

$$q_i^B(q_j) = \frac{\alpha_i - m_i - \gamma_{ij} q_j}{2\beta_i}. \tag{4}$$

Consider now the situation where the current output $q_i(t)$ is different from the best response $q_i^B(q_j)$ as given in (4). The firm then needs to have an adjustment process that will bring its production to the desired level. Here we consider an adjustment process that is given by a logistic equation:

$$\frac{dq_i(t)}{dt} = k_i (q_i^B(q_j) - q_i(t)) q_i(t) \tag{5}$$

where k_i controls the speed of the adjustment.[16] The larger k is, the steeper the firm has to ramp or reduce its current output to meet the desired level.

Given the adjustment process above, the resulting dynamical equations become:

$$\frac{dq_i(t)}{dt} = k_i q_i(t) (M_i - q_i(t) - c_{ij} q_j(t)) \tag{6}$$

where

$$M_i = \frac{\alpha_i - m_i}{2\beta_i}$$
$$\tag{7}$$
$$c_{ij} = \frac{\gamma_{ij}}{2\beta_i}.$$

Equation (6) is formally equivalent to the Lotka-Volterra competitive equations. The maximum output of firm i will be realized when firm j ceases to produce (i.e. $q_j = 0$). This monopoly output M_i is just the carrying capacity of the firm and is proportional to the firm's net advantage $(\alpha_i - m_i)$. One can extract as well the competition coefficient c_{ij} and is proportional to the differentiation of the products (γ_{ij}).

3. Critical Transitions

Given the dynamics above, we now investigate the equilibrium states and transitions near them. The model above has the following equilibrium points, eigenvalues and stability conditions.

Table 1. Equilibria, eigenvalues and stability conditions of the model.

Equilibrium Points (q_1^*, q_2^*)	Eigenvalues	Stable if
$(0,0)$	$\lambda_1 = k_1 M_1; \lambda_2 = k_2 M_2$	Never
$(M_1, 0)$	$\lambda_1 = -k_1 M_1$	$c_{21} > \frac{M_2}{M_1}$
	$\lambda_2 = -k_2 (c_{21} M_1 - M_2)$	
$(0, M_2)$	$\lambda_1 = -k_2 M_2$	$c_{12} > \frac{M_1}{M_2}$
	$\lambda_2 = -k_1 (c_{12} M_2 - M_1)$	
$\left(\frac{M_1 - c_{12} M_2}{1 - c_{12} c_{21}}, \frac{M_2 - c_{21} M_1}{1 - c_{12} c_{21}} \right)$	$\lambda_\pm = \frac{-(a+b) \pm \sqrt{(a+b)^2 - 4(1 - c_{12} c_{21})ab}}{2}$	$c_{12} c_{21} < 1$
	$a = k_1 q_1^*; b - k_2 q_2^*$	

The first equilibrium point is the trivial case where both firms do not produce and this condition is never stable as the eigenvalues are both positive. The next two results in the persistence of one firm and the demise of the other. This condition is stable if the impact of one firm on the other, as given by the competition coefficient, is larger than the ratio between the firms' monopoly output. The last equilibrium point pertain to the coexistence of the firms. This is stable if the impact of each firm is less than the ratio of their monopoly outputs.

Now we investigate the transition from one dynamical state to another and see how the equilibrium values change as one parameter is varied. Suppose changes in the business condition alters the advantage of firm 1 but have no effect on firm 2. This can be a change in its quality or cost structure (or both) resulting in a change in M_1. For M_1 very small compared to M_2, firm 2 would eventually monopolize the market. However as M_1 improves it would be possible to coexist with firm 2. The value of M_1 that would allow this and the type of coexistence depends on the kind of competition.

For $c_{12} c_{21} > 1$, a path dependent hysteresis-like phenomenon occurs. For smaller values of M_1, firm 2 would be the only one left in the long-term evolution of the competition. However, past $c_{12} M_2$ it will trade places with firm 2 – firm 1 now monopolizing the market. Reversing the direction, for high values of M_1, firm 1 will be the monopoly until it decreases below M_2/c_{21} where firm 2 becomes the monopoly. In between M_2/c_{21} and $c_{12} M_2$, an unstable coexistence (dotted lines) prevails with the outcome depending on their initial conditions. These features are shown in Figure 1.a.

For $c_{12} c_{21} < 1$, a stable coexistence occurs when $M_1 > c_{12} M_2$. Improving beyond M_2/c_{21} results in firm 1 monopolizing the market. The graph of the equilibrium values as a function of M_1 is depicted in Figure 1.b.

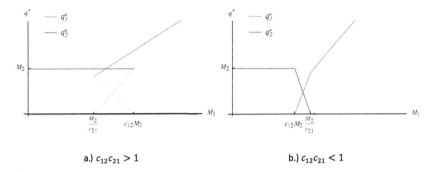

a.) $c_{12}c_{21} > 1$ b.) $c_{12}c_{21} < 1$

Fig. 1.   (Color online) Equilibrium values as a function of M_1 for firm 1 and firm 2.

4. Critical Slowing Down

Given the transitions above, of interest would be to find a way the transitions can be anticipated. To go about this, we take a look at the characteristic return time required for the system from an initial state $q_i(t_o)$ to a later state $q_i(t_f)$ as a function of the monopoly output M_1. From (6), this would be given by:

$$T_i(M_i) = \int_{t_o}^{t_f} dt = \frac{1}{k_i} \int_{q_i}^{q_f} \frac{dq_i}{q_i(M_i - q_i - c_{ij}q_j)}. \tag{8}$$

For instance, for M_1 smaller than $c_{12}M_2$, the equilibrium state would have $q_1^* = 0$ and $q_2^* = M_2$. However as M_1 increases we can estimate the return time from a very small value ε to a quantity q_f

$$T_1(M_1) = \frac{1}{k_1} \int_{\varepsilon}^{q_f} \frac{dq_i}{q_1(M_1 - q_1 - c_{12}M_2)}$$

$$= \frac{1}{k_1(M_1 - c_{12}M_2)} \ln\left(\frac{\varepsilon(q_f - M_1 + c_{12}M_2)}{q_f(\varepsilon - M_1 + c_{12}M_2)}\right). \tag{9}$$

On the other side of the critical point, the equilibrium state would be $(q_1^*, q_2^*) = \left(\frac{M_1 - c_{12}M_2}{1 - c_{12}c_{21}}, \frac{M_2 - c_{21}M_1}{1 - c_{12}c_{21}}\right)$. As such coming from $q_1^* + \varepsilon$ to q_f would take about:

$$T_1(M_1) = \frac{1}{k_1} \int_{q_1^* + \varepsilon}^{q_f} \frac{dq_i}{q_1(M_1 - q_1 - c_{12}q_2^*)}$$

$$= \frac{1}{k_1(M_1 - c_{12}q_2^*)} \ln\left(\frac{(q_1^* + \varepsilon)(q_f - M_1 + c_{12}q_2^*)}{q_f(q_1^* + \varepsilon - M_1 + c_{12}q_2^*)}\right). \tag{10}$$

Plotting the return time as a function of M_1 yields the graph in Figure 2.

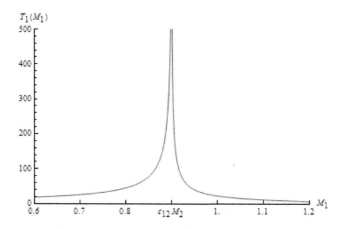

Fig. 2. Return time as a function of M_1. ($M_2 = 12$, $c_{12} = c_{21} = 075$, $q_f = 075$, $\varepsilon = 0001$).

Evident in the graph is the rapid increase in the return time as the control parameter M_1 approaches the critical point $c_{12}M_2$. This critical slowing down on both directions comes before the actual critical transition.

A more general process of anticipating critical transitions using the concept of critical slowing has been developed.[17] The characteristic return time is obtained from the recovery rate ρ which is just the absolute value of the real part of the dominant eigenvalue. For instance, consider the transition from $(M_1, 0)$ to (M_2) for the case $c_{12}c_{21} > 1$. From the eigenvalues in Table 1.

$$\rho = |Re(\lambda_{\text{dominant}})| = \min\left(k_1M_1, k_2\left(c_{21}M_1 - M_2\right)\right). \tag{11}$$

Using Eq. (11), if $k_1M_1 < k_2\left(c_{21}M_1 - M_2\right)$ then $\rho_1 = k_1M_1$.[18] This recovery rate would be true for $M_1 > k_2M_2/(k_2c_{21} - k_1)$. Otherwise, $\rho_1 = k_2\left(c_{21}M_1 - M_2\right)$. As such as the control parameter M_1 decreases, the recovery rate is decreasing as well, slowing down and becoming zero at the critical transition M_2/c_{21}. Similarly, for the state (M_2) the recovery rate $\rho_2 = k_2M_2$ for $M_1 < M_2(k_1c_{12} - k_2)/k_1$ and $\rho_2 = k_1\left(c_{12}M_2 - M_1\right)$ otherwise. We then can superimpose the recovery rates to the plot of the equilibrium values as shown in Figure 3.

Evident in the figure is the discontinuous change in the recovery rate prior to the critical transitions in the equilibrium values. For instance, for firm 2 the recovery rate has changed at $(c_{12} - k_2/k_1)M_2$ whereas the abrupt change in its equilibrium value happened at $c_{12}M_2$. One can then measure the absolute change in the control parameter M_1 before the critical transition sets in, which in this case would be $(k_2/k_1)M_2 = r_2M_2$ where r_j is the relative speed of adjustment of firm j to firm i. The higher r_2 is, the greater k_2 is compared to k_1, and the "sooner" the early warning could be.

Similarly for firm 1, the abrupt end of its decline can be forewarned by its recovery rate. Before it declines to M_2/c_{21}, the recovery rate has undergone a discontinuous change at $M_2/(c_{21} - k_1/k_2)$. As such a decline of $k_1M_2/k_2c_{21}(c_{21} - k_1/k_2)$ more

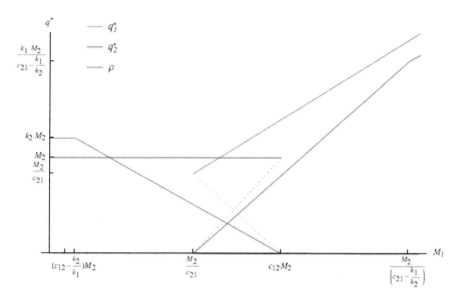

Fig. 3. (Color online) Equilibrium values (q_1^*, q_2^*) and recovery rates ρ for $c_{12}c_{21} > 1$.

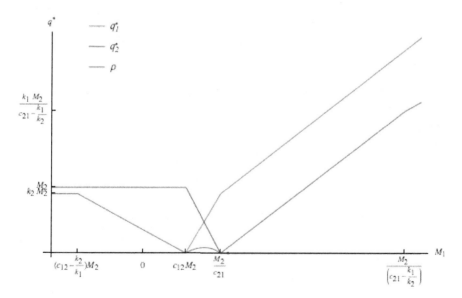

Fig. 4. (Color online) Equilibrium values (q_1^*, q_2^*) and recovery rates ρ for $c_{12}c_{21} < 1$.

will bring it to the threshold of the critical transition. Rewriting to $r_1 M_2 / c_{21}(c_{21} - r_1)$, the critical transition can be forewarned earlier if the competitive impact of firm 1 on 2 is low (i.e. low c_{21}) or the relative speed of adjustment r_1 is large ($k_1 > k_2$).

For the case of $c_{12}c_{21} < 1$, the presence or absence of a region for an early warning signal becomes more defined. Similar to the case of $c_{12}c_{21} > 1$, the discontinuous transitions of the recovery rate occur at $(c_{12}-r_2)M_2$ for firm 2 and at $r_1 M_2/(c_{21}-r_1)$ for firm 1 as shown in Figure 4. However, the presence of one precludes the other as an early warning signal as $r_2 < c_{12}$ automatically means that $c_{21} - r_1 < 0$. And $c_{21} > r_1$ implies $r_2 > c_{12}$ as illustrated in the figure below (i.e $(c_{12} - r_2) M_2 < 0$). As such, only the firm whose relative speed of adjustment is $r_i < c_{ji}i \neq j$ can have an early warning from its recovery rate.

5. Conclusion

Of interest from the preceding results is the role that the relative speed of adjustment $r_i = k_i/k_j$ plays in the presence or absence of an early warning signal. For r_1 very large, $c_{21} - r_1$ becomes negative and the discontinuous change of the recovery rate occurs at a negative monopoly output of firm 1 which is not realistic. Similarly, for large r_2, $c_{12} - r_2$ can become negative and firm 2 loses an early warning signal. As such, only at regions where $r_i < c_{ji}$ or $k_i < c_{ji}k_j$ does an early warning signal for both firms makes sense. Otherwise, the monopoly output shifts to negative and hence no longer feasible.

As such, it is possible to use the concept of critical slowing down to provide early warning to the critical transitions in a dynamic duopoly. The extent of the early warning depends on the monopoly output, competition coefficient and relative speed of adjustment. If the monopoly output is large, because, for instance of large firm advantage, the farther the warning is from a critical transition. The smaller the impact of the competition is, that is the smaller the competition coefficient, the more time one is forewarned. And the larger the relative speed of adjustment is, the sooner is the early warning.

References

1. M. Scheffer, J. Bascompte, W.A. Brock, V. Brovkin, S.R. Carpenter and V. Dakos, Early-warning signals for critical transitions, *Nature* **461**, 53(2009).
2. M. Scheffer, S.R. Carpenter, T.M. Lenton, J. Bascompte, W. Brock, V. Dakos, J. van de Koppel, I.A. van de Leemput, S.A. Levin, E.H. van Nes, M. Pascual and J. Vandermeer, Anticipating Critical Transitions, *Science* **338**, 344(2012).
3. C. Wissel, A universal law of characteristic return time near thresholds, *Oecologia* **65**, 101(1984).
4. J.R. Tredicce, G.L. Lippia, P. Mandel, B. Charasse, A. Chevalier and B. Picque, Critical slowing down at a bifurcation, *American Journal of Physics* **72**, 799(2004).
5. J. Lim and B.I. Epureanu, Forecasting a class of bifurcations: Theory and experiment, *Physical Review E* **83**, 016203(2011).
6. C. Diks and C. Hommes, Early warning signals for critical transitions in finance, (Royal Economic Society Annual Conference, London, 2013).
7. D. Sornette, Critical market crashes, *Physics Reports* **378**, 1(2003).
8. R.E. Farmer, The stock market crash of 2008 caused the Great Recession: Theory and evidence, *Journal of Economic Dynamics and Control* **36**, 693(2012).

9. J.W. Friedman, *Oligopoly Theory*, (Cambridge University Press, Cambridge, MA 1983).
10. M. Kopel, Simple and complex adjustment dynamics in Cournot duopoly models, *Chaos, Solitons and Fractals* **7**, 2031(1996).
11. D. Rand, Exotic phenomena in games and duopoly models, *Journal of Mathematical Economics* **5**, 173(1978).
12. J. Tirole, *The theory of industrial organization* (MIT Press, Cambridge, MA, 1988).
13. W. Mas-Collel, M.D. Green and J.R. Green, *Microeconomic Theory* (Oxford University Press, Oxford, 1995).
14. N. Singh and X. Vives, Price and Quantity Competition in a Differentiated Duopoly, *The RAND Journal of Economics* **15**, 546(1984).
15. A.A. Cournot, *Researches into the Mathematical Principles of the Theory of Wealth* (Kelley, New York, 1960).
16. M.O. Escobido, Product interactions and industry shakeout, *International Journal of Modern Physics: Conference Series* **17**, 104(2012).
17. E.H. van Nes and M. Scheffer, Slow recovery from perturbations as a generic indicator of a nearby catastrophic shift, *American Naturalist* **169**, 738(2007).
18. R.A. Chisholm and E. Filotas, Critical slowing down as an indicator of transitions in two-species models, *Journal of Theoretical Biology* **257**, 142(2009).

7th Jagna International Workshop (2014)
International Journal of Modern Physics: Conference Series
Vol. 36 (2015) 1560013 (8 pages)
© The Author
DOI: 10.1142/S2010194515600137

World Scientific
www.worldscientific.com

Measuring efficiency of international crude oil markets:
A multifractality approach

H. M. Niere

Economics Department, Mindanao State University,
Marawi City, 9700, Philippines
hmniere@gmail.com
www.msumain.edu.ph

Published 2 January 2015

The three major international crude oil markets are treated as complex systems and their multifractal properties are explored. The study covers daily prices of Brent crude, OPEC reference basket and West Texas Intermediate (WTI) crude from January 2, 2003 to January 2, 2014. A multifractal detrended fluctuation analysis (MFDFA) is employed to extract the generalized Hurst exponents in each of the time series. The generalized Hurst exponent is used to measure the degree of multifractality which in turn is used to quantify the efficiency of the three international crude oil markets. To identify whether the source of multifractality is long-range correlations or broad fat-tail distributions, shuffled data and surrogated data corresponding to each of the time series are generated. Shuffled data are obtained by randomizing the order of the price returns data. This will destroy any long-range correlation of the time series. Surrogated data is produced using the Fourier-Detrended Fluctuation Analysis (F-DFA). This is done by randomizing the phases of the price returns data in Fourier space. This will normalize the distribution of the time series. The study found that for the three crude oil markets, there is a strong dependence of the generalized Hurst exponents with respect to the order of fluctuations. This shows that the daily price time series of the markets under study have signs of multifractality. Using the degree of multifractality as a measure of efficiency, the results show that WTI is the most efficient while OPEC is the least efficient market. This implies that OPEC has the highest likelihood to be manipulated among the three markets. This reflects the fact that Brent and WTI is a very competitive market hence, it has a higher level of complexity compared against OPEC, which has a large monopoly power. Comparing with shuffled data and surrogated data, the findings suggest that for all the three crude oil markets, the multifractality is mainly due to long-range correlations.

Keywords: Multifractality; Hurst exponents; oil markets; efficiency.

1. Introduction

Fractals as introduced by Mandelbrot[1-2] describe geometric patterns with large degree of self-similarities at all scales. The smaller piece of a pattern can be said to be a reduced-form image of a larger piece. This characteristic is used to measure fractal dimensions as a fraction rather than an integer. Some examples of fractal shapes are rugged coastlines, mountain heights, cloud outlines, river tributaries, tree branches, blood vessels, cracks, wave turbulences and chaotic motions. However, there are self-similar patterns that involve multiple scaling rules which are not sufficiently described by a single fractal dimension but by a spectrum of fractal dimensions instead. Generalizing this single dimension into multiple dimensions differentiates multifractal from fractals discussed earlier. To distinguish multifractal from single fractal, the term monofractal is used for single fractal in this paper. Among the natural systems that have been observed to have a multifractal property are earthquakes,[3] heart rate variability[4] and neural activities.[5]

Mandelbrot[6] introduced multifractal models to study economic and financial time series in order to address the shortcomings of traditional models such as fractional Brownian motion and GARCH processes which are not appropriate with the stylized facts of the said time series such as long-memory and fat-tails in volatility. Further studies confirmed multifractality in stock market indices,[7-16] foreign exchange rates[17-20] and interest rates,[21] to name a few. As a consequence, many studies have now used the properties of multifractality in forecasting models.[22-24] These models are at least as good as, and in some cases, perform better using out-of-sample forecast compared to traditional models. One added advantage of these models is their being parsimonious.

This paper investigates the presence and compares the degree of multifractality of the daily prices of crude oil of the three major international crude oil markets namely the Brent crude, OPEC reference basket and West Texas Intermediate (WTI) crude from January 2, 2003 to January 2, 2014. The Brent crude is sourced from the North Sea and is the main European oil market; OPEC is mainly sourced from the Middle East; and WTI is the benchmark used in Chicago and New York mercantile exchange. Furthermore, since multifractality can be due to long-range correlations or due to broad fat-tail distributions, this paper identifies which of the two factors dominates the multifractality of the daily crude prices time series of the said markets. The paper is arranged as follows. Methodology is discussed in Section 2. Data are described in Section 3. Presentation of results is in Section 4. Finally, the paper concludes in Section 5.

2. Methodology

In measuring multifractality, the paper uses the method of Multifractal Detrended Fluctuation Analysis (MFDFA) as outlined in Kantelhardt *et al.*[25] Matlab codes used are based in Ihlen.[26] The procedure is summarized in the following steps.

(1) Given a time series u_i, $i = 1, \ldots, N$, where N is the length, create a profile $Y(k) = \sum_{i=1}^{k} u_i - \bar{u}$, $k = 1, \ldots, N$, where $\bar{u}$ is the mean of u.

(2) Divide the profile $Y(k)$ into $N_s = N/s$ non-overlapping segment of length s. Since N is not generally a multiple of s, in order for the remainder part of the series to be included, this step is repeated starting at the end of the series moving backwards. Thus, a total of $2N_s$ segments are produced.

(3) Generate $Y_s(i) = Y_s[(v-1)s+i]$ for each segment $v = 1, \ldots, N_s$, and $Y_s(i) = Y_s[N - (v - N_s)s + i]$ for each segment $v = N_s + 1, \ldots, 2N_s$.

(4) Compute the variance of $Y_s(i)$ as $F_s^2(v) = \frac{1}{s} \sum_{i=1}^{s} [Y_s(i) - Y_v(i)]^2$, where $Y_v(i)$ is the mth order fitting polynomial in the vth segment.

(5) Obtain the qth order fluctuation function by

$$
F_q(s) = \left\{ \frac{1}{2N_s} \sum_{v=1}^{2N_s} [F_s^2(v)]^{q/2} \right\}^{1/q}.
$$

If the time series are long-range correlated then $F_q(s)$ is distributed as power laws, $F_q(s) \sim s^{h(q)}$. The exponent $h(q)$ is called as the generalized Hurst exponent. When $h(q) = 0.5$, this implies that the fluctuations are just random walks.

For monofractals, the Hurst exponent is a constant equal to $h(2)$. The closer the value of $h(2)$ to 0.5, the more closely the time series mimics random walk. Hence, market efficiency can be measured by the distance of $h(2)$ from 0.5. For multifractals however, $h(q)$ varies with q. Thus, a spectrum of $h(q)$ values implies the presence of multifractality.

The degree of multifractality can be quantified as $|\Delta h| = h(q_{min}) - h(q_{min})$. Moreover, the higher the degree of multifractality, the lower the market efficiency.[23]

To identify whether the multifractality is due to long-range correlations or is due to broad fat-tail distributions, shuffled data and surrogated data are generated. In the spirit of Zunino *et al.*,[11] 100 different shuffled time series and surrogated time series are produced to reduce statistical errors. Shuffling the data will remove the long-range correlation in the time series. It is done by randomizing the order of the original data. The multifractality due to long-range correlation can be computed as $h_c = \Delta h - \Delta h_f$ where the index f refers to shuffled data.

Surrogated data is produced by randomizing the phases of original data in Fourier space. This will make the data to have normal distribution. The multifractality due to broad fat-tail distributions can be measured as $h_d = \Delta h - \Delta h_r$ where the index r refers to surrogated data.

3. Data

The daily crude oil prices of the Brent crude, OPEC reference basket and WTI crude from January 2, 2003 to January 2, 2014 are used for a total of 2788, 2839 and 2765 observations respectively. The number of observations differs for the three markets because the number of business trading days also differs due to national holidays and other idiosyncracies. Daily price data for OPEC reference basket has been downloaded from the OPEC online database website: http://www.opec.org/opec_web/en/data_graphs/40.htm. The daily price data for Brent and WTI crude was downloaded from the website of the U.S. Energy Information Administration: http://www.eia.gov/dnav/pet/pet_pri_spt_s1_d.htm.

4. Results

Figures 1 to 3 show the plots of the daily crude prices, the daily returns, and the associated shuffled and surrogated time series of daily returns for Brent crude, OPEC reference basket and WTI crude respectively. The original daily returns and the shuffled time series show some extreme fluctuations which is a sign of having fat-tail distribution. The surrogated time series do not have extreme fluctuation, a characteristic of a normal distribution.

In doing the MFDFA procedure, $m = 3$ is used as the order of polynomial fit in Step 3. The length s varies from 20 to $N/4$ with a step of 4 as suggested in Kantelhardt *et al.*[25] Finally, q runs from -10 to 10 with a step of 0.5. Figure 2 presents the generalized Hurst exponents for the original returns, shuffled returns and surrogated returns. For monofractals, the Hurst exponent is independent of q which is also equal to the generalized Hurst exponents of multifractals at$q = 2$, that

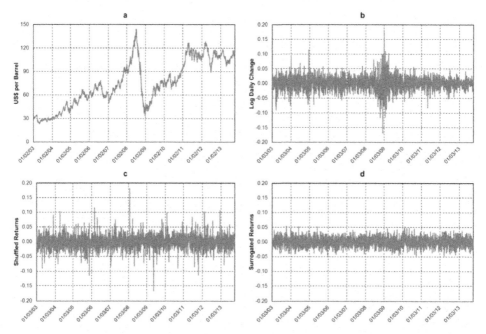

Fig. 1. (Color online) Plots of the (a) daily Brent crude oil price, (b) its daily returns, (c) shuffled time series, and (d) surrogated time series.

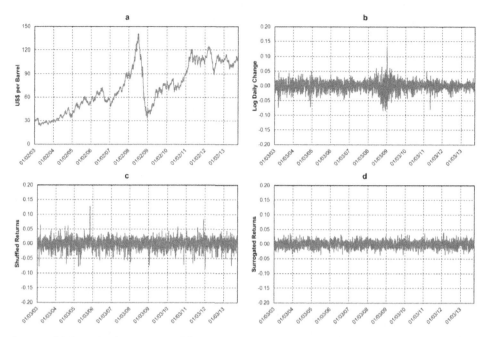

Fig. 2.   (Color online) Plots of the (a) daily OPEC crude oil price, (b) its daily returns, (c) shuffled time series, and (d) surrogated time series.

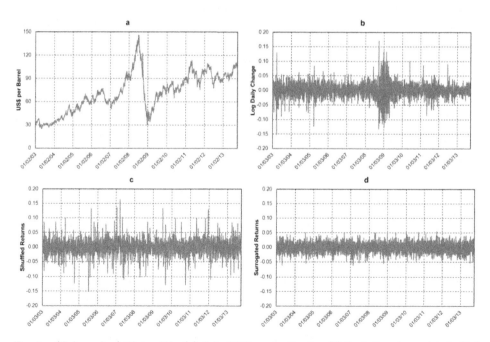

Fig. 3.   (Color online) Plots of the (a) daily WTI crude oil price, (b) its daily returns, (c) shuffled time series, and (d) surrogated time series.

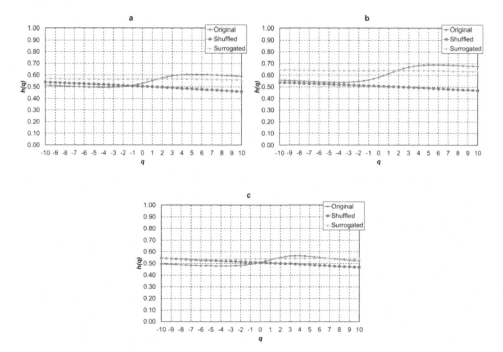

Fig. 4.   (Color online) Generalized Hurst exponent, $h(q)$, as a function of q for the original, shuffled and surrogated daily returns for (a) Brent crude, (b) OPEC reference basket, and (c) WTI crude.

is, $h(2)$. In other words, monofractals have only one single Hurst exponent which is $h(2)$ regardless of the value of q. In contrast, multifractals have a spectrum of generalized Hurst exponents which vary depending upon the value of q. It is noted in Figure 2 that for the daily returns time series, $h(q)$ is dependent upon q. As q increases, $h(q)$ decreases. This is a confirmation that the daily crude price time series of the three international crude oil markets are indeed multifractals. This suggests that monofractal models are not appropriate for this time series.

Table 1 presents the generalized Hurst exponents, $h(q)$ with values of q ranging from -10 to 10 for the original return time series, shuffled and surrogated time series. Since for all the three markets, we have $|h_c| > |h_d|$. This means that the multifractality is mainly due to long-range correlations.

Using $|\Delta h|$ as a measure of efficiency, we can conclude that WTI is the most efficient while OPEC is the least efficient market. This implies that OPEC has the highest likelihood to be manipulated among the three markets. This reflects the fact that Brent and WTI is a very competitive market hence, it has a higher level of complexity compared against OPEC, which has a large monopoly power.

Table 1. Generalized Hurst exponents, $h(q)$ with $q = -10$ to 10.

q	Brent			OPEC			WTI		
	Original	Shuffled	Surrogated	Original	Shuffled	Surrogated	Original	Shuffled	Surrogated
-10	0.4991	0.5427	0.5750	0.5496	0.5337	0.6397	0.4928	0.5410	0.5380
-9	0.4974	0.5412	0.5742	0.5477	0.5322	0.6387	0.4913	0.5393	0.5375
-8	0.4957	0.5397	0.5734	0.5458	0.5307	0.6377	0.4897	0.5374	0.5369
-7	0.4940	0.5381	0.5727	0.5439	0.5291	0.6367	0.4882	0.5355	0.5365
-6	0.4923	0.5365	0.5720	0.5420	0.5276	0.6358	0.4867	0.5336	0.5361
-5	0.4907	0.5349	0.5713	0.5401	0.5260	0.6350	0.4852	0.5316	0.5357
-4	0.4892	0.5333	0.5707	0.5382	0.5244	0.6342	0.4837	0.5296	0.5354
-3	0.4878	0.5316	0.5702	0.5365	0.5228	0.6334	0.4823	0.5276	0.5353
-2	0.4865	0.5300	0.5697	0.5349	0.5212	0.6328	0.4810	0.5255	0.5352
-1	0.4854	0.5284	0.5692	0.5334	0.5197	0.6322	0.4798	0.5234	0.5352
0	0.4846	0.5268	0.5689	0.5322	0.5181	0.6318	0.4788	0.5213	0.5353
1	0.4841	0.5251	0.5686	0.5313	0.5165	0.6315	0.4781	0.5191	0.5356
2	0.4841	0.5235	0.5684	0.5309	0.5150	0.6312	0.4778	0.5170	0.5360
3	0.4846	0.5219	0.5682	0.5312	0.5135	0.6311	0.4779	0.5148	0.5365
4	0.4860	0.5203	0.5681	0.5322	0.5120	0.6312	0.4786	0.5127	0.5371
5	0.4883	0.5187	0.5681	0.5343	0.5105	0.6313	0.4801	0.5105	0.5378
6	0.4917	0.5171	0.5682	0.5379	0.5091	0.6316	0.4826	0.5083	0.5387
7	0.4967	0.5156	0.5683	0.5432	0.5076	0.6320	0.4864	0.5061	0.5396
8	0.5034	0.5140	0.5685	0.5508	0.5062	0.6324	0.4919	0.5038	0.5406
9	0.5122	0.5123	0.5687	0.5611	0.5047	0.6329	0.4993	0.5016	0.5416
10	0.5231	0.5107	0.5689	0.5743	0.5032	0.6335	0.5087	0.4993	0.5427
Δh	0.5360	0.5090	0.5691	0.5904	0.5017	0.6341	0.5200	0.4970	0.5437
	$h_c = -0.1787$		$h_d = -0.1179$	$h_c = -0.2053$		$h_d = -0.1485$	$h_c = -0.1195$		$h_d = -0.0226$

References

1. B.B. Mandelbrot, *Fractals: Form, Chance and Dimension* (W. H. Freeman and Co., San Francisco, 1977).
2. B.B. Mandelbrot, *The Fractal Geometry of Nature* (W. H. Freeman and Co., New York, 1982).
3. G. Parisi and U. Frisch, Turbulence and Predictability in Geophysical Fluid Dynamics and Climate Dynamics, in *Proc. of the International School "Enrico Fermi"*, (North-Holland, Amsterdam, Netherlands, 1985).
4. A.L. Goldberger, L.A. Amaral, J.M. Hausdorff, P.C. Ivanov, C. K. Peng and H.E. Stanley, Fractal dynamics in physiology: Alterations with disease and aging, in *Proc. Natl. Acad. Sci.* (2002), p. 2466.
5. Y. Zheng, J.B. Gao, J.C. Sanchez, J.C. Principe and M.S. Okun, *Phys. Lett.* **A 344**, 253 (2005).
6. B.B. Mandelbrot, *Fractals and Scaling in Finance* (Springer, New York, 1997).
7. H. Katsuragi, *Phys.* **A 278**, 275 (2000).
8. Z.-Q. Jiang and W.-X. Zhou, *Phys.* **A 387**, 4881 (2008).
9. X. Sun, H. Chen, Z. Wu and Y. Yuan, *Phys.* **A 291**, 553 (2001).
10. P. Oswiecimka, J. Kwapien, S. Drozdz, A. Z. Gorski and R. Rak, *Act. Phys. Polo.* **B 37**, 3083 (2006).
11. L. Zunino, A. Figliola, B.M. Tabak, D.G. Pérez, M. Garavaglia and O.A. Rosso, *Chaos, Solitons & Fractals* **41**, 2331 (2009).
12. L. Zunino, B.M. Tabak, A. Figliola, D.G. Pérez, M. Garavaglia and O.A. Rosso, *Phys.* **A 387**, 6558 (2008).
13. C.-T. Lye and C.-W. Hooy, *Int. J. of Econ. and Mgt.* **6**(2), pp 278–294, 2012.
14. X. Lu, J. Tian, Y. Zhou and Z. Li, *Working Papers 2012-08* (Department of Economics, Auckland University of Technology, 2012).
15. Y. Yuan, X.-T. Zhuang and X. Jin, *Phys.* **A 388**, 2189 (2009).
16. W. Hui, Z. Zongfang and X. Luojie, *Mgt. Sci. and Engg.* **6**, 21 (2012).
17. N. Vandewalle and M. Ausloos, *Eur. Phys. J.* **B 4**, 257 (1998).
18. P. Norouzzadeh and B. Rahmani, *Phys.* **A 367**, 328 (2006).
19. G. Oh, C. Eom, S. Havlin, W.-S. Jung, F. Wang, H.E. Stanley and S. Kim, *Eur. Phys. J.* **B 85**, 214 (2012).
20. T. Ioan, P. Anita and C. Razvan, *Ann. of Fac. of Econ.* **1**, 784 (Faculty of Economics, University of Oradea, 2012).
21. D.O. Cajueiro and B.M. Tabak, *Phys.* **A 373**, 603 (2007).
22. T. Lux, *Economics Working Paper No.* 2003, 13 (Department of Economics, Christian-Albrechts-Universität Kiel, 2003).
23. T. Lux, *Economics Working Paper No.* 2006, 17 (Department of Economics, Christian-Albrechts-Universität Kiel, 2006).
24. T. Lux, L. Morales-Arias and C. Sattarhoff, *Kiel Working Paper* 1737, (Kiel Institute for the World Economy, 2011).
25. J.W. Kantelhardt, S.A. Zschiegner, E. Koscielny-Bunde, S. Havlin, A. Bunde and H.E. Stanley, *Phys.* **A 316**, 87 (2002).
26. E.A.F. Ihlen, *Front Physiol* **3**, 141 (2012).

7th Jagna International Workshop (2014)
International Journal of Modern Physics: Conference Series
Vol. 36 (2015) 1560014 (5 pages)
© The Authors
DOI: 10.1142/S2010194515600149

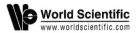

Space-fractional Schrödinger equation for a quadrupolar triple Dirac-δ potential: Central Dirac-δ well and barrier cases

Jeffrey D. Tare* and Jose Perico H. Esguerra

*National Institute of Physics, University of the Philippines–Diliman,
Quezon City 1101, Philippines*
*jeffreytare@gmail.com
www.nip.upd.edu.ph*

Published 2 January 2015

We solve the space-fractional Schrödinger equation for a quadrupolar triple Dirac-δ (QTD-δ) potential for all energies using the momentum-space approach. For the $E < 0$ solution, we consider two cases, i.e., when the strengths of the potential are $V_0 > 0$ (QTD-δ potential with central Dirac-δ well) and $V_0 < 0$ (QTD-δ potential with central Dirac-δ barrier) and derive expressions satisfied by the bound-state energy. For all fractional orders α considered, we find that there is one eigenenergy when $V_0 > 0$, and there are two eigenenergies when $V_0 < 0$. We also obtain both bound- and scattering-state ($E > 0$) wave functions and express them in terms of Fox's H-function.

Keywords: Fractional quantum mechanics; space-fractional Schrödinger equation; quadrupolar triple Dirac-δ potential; Fox's H-function.

1. Introduction

Applications of fractional quantum mechanics (FQM) developed by Laskin[1,2] via constructing fractional path integral over paths of Lévy flights have gained interest over the past 13 years. The formulation offers generalization of some results obtained in the standard quantum mechanics (SQM). One of its interesting applications is to delta potentials.[3] Here we present another application of FQM by considering a quadrupolar triple Dirac-δ (QTD-δ) potential in one dimension, which was first analyzed by Patil[4] in the framework of SQM.

The time-independent space-fractional Schrödinger equation (TISFSE) in the position representation reads[2]

$$D_\alpha(-\hbar^2\Delta)^{\alpha/2}\psi(x) + V(x)\psi(x) = E\psi(x), \quad 1 < \alpha \leq 2, \tag{1}$$

where D_α is the generalized quantum diffusion coefficient [$D_2 = 1/(2m)$ with m being the mass of the particle], $\psi(x)$ is the wave function, $V(x)$ is the potential, E

is the energy, and $(-\hbar^2 \Delta)^{\alpha/2}$ is the quantum Riesz fractional derivative:

$$(-\hbar^2 \Delta)^{\alpha/2} \psi(x) = \frac{1}{2\pi\hbar} \int_{-\infty}^{\infty} dp \, e^{ipx/\hbar} |p|^{\alpha} \int_{-\infty}^{\infty} e^{-ipx'/\hbar} \psi(x') dx'. \qquad (2)$$

In the momentum representation the TISFSE can be expressed as[3]

$$D_\alpha |p|^\alpha \tilde{\psi}(p) + \frac{(\tilde{V} * \tilde{\psi})(p)}{2\pi\hbar} = E\tilde{\psi}(p), \qquad (3)$$

where $\tilde{\psi}(p) = \int_{-\infty}^{\infty} e^{-ipx/\hbar} \psi(x) dx$ is the Fourier transform of $\psi(x)$, with the inverse transform $\psi(x) = (2\pi\hbar)^{-1} \int_{-\infty}^{\infty} e^{ipx/\hbar} \tilde{\psi}(p) dp$, and $(\tilde{V} * \tilde{\psi})(p)$ is the convolution of $\tilde{V}(p)$ and $\tilde{\psi}(p)$: $(\tilde{V} * \tilde{\psi})(p) = \int_{-\infty}^{\infty} \tilde{V}(p - p') \tilde{\psi}(p') dp'$. In the next section we solve Eq. (1) for a QTD-δ potential using the momentum-space approach.

2. QTD-δ Potential and Solutions to the TISFSE

The interaction between an electron and a symmetric linear triatomic molecule can be modeled using the potential[4] $V(x) = V_0[\delta(x + a) - 2\delta(x) + \delta(x - a)]$, where V_0 is the strength and a is the spacing between the atoms. Its Fourier transform and convolution with $\tilde{\psi}(p)$ are given, respectively, by $\tilde{V}(p) = V_0(e^{iap/\hbar} - 2 + e^{-iap/\hbar})$ and $(\tilde{V} * \tilde{\psi})(p) = V_0[e^{iap/\hbar} C_0(a) - 2C_1(0) + e^{-iap/\hbar} C_2(a)]$, where the constants are defined as $C_0(a) = C_2(-a) = \int_{-\infty}^{\infty} e^{-iap'/\hbar} \tilde{\psi}(p') dp'$ and $C_1(0) = \int_{-\infty}^{\infty} \tilde{\psi}(p') dp'$. Substituting the expression for $(\tilde{V} * \tilde{\psi})(p)$ in Eq. (3), we obtain an expression for $\tilde{\psi}(p)$:

$$\tilde{\psi}(p) = \frac{-\gamma_\alpha}{(|p|^\alpha - E/D_\alpha)} [e^{iap/\hbar} C_0(a) - 2C_1(0) + e^{-iap/\hbar} C_2(a)], \qquad (4)$$

with $\gamma_\alpha = V_0/2\pi\hbar D_\alpha$. Below we solve the TISFSE for two separate cases, namely, $E < 0$ and $E > 0$.

Case I: $E < 0$. For this case, let us first consider $V_0 > 0$ (central Dirac-δ well case) and define $\lambda^\alpha = -E/D_\alpha$ ($\lambda > 0$). Equation (4) then becomes $\tilde{\psi}(p) = -\gamma_\alpha(|p|^\alpha + \lambda^\alpha)^{-1}[e^{iap/\hbar} C_0(a) - 2C_1(0) + e^{-iap/\hbar} C_2(a)]$. When we use this expression to find C_0, C_1, C_2, an equation satisfied by bound-state energy can be derived, namely, $R\epsilon^{\alpha-1} A(\epsilon) = R^3 \epsilon^{3(\alpha-1)} - B(\epsilon)$, where $\epsilon = a\lambda/\hbar$, $R = 2\pi\hbar^\alpha D_\alpha/(a^{\alpha-1} V_0)$, $A(\epsilon) = 3T^2(0) - 4T^2(\epsilon) + T^2(2\epsilon)$, $B(\epsilon) = 2\{T(0)[T^2(0) - 2T^2(\epsilon) - T^2(2\epsilon)] + 2T^2(\epsilon)T(2\epsilon)\}$, and $T(y) = 2\int_0^\infty \cos(yq)(q^\alpha + 1)^{-1} dq$ ($q = p/\lambda$). Figure 1 shows plots of the functions $f(\alpha, \epsilon) = R\epsilon^{\alpha-1} A(\epsilon)$ and $h(\alpha, \epsilon) = R^3 \epsilon^{3(\alpha-1)} - B(\epsilon)$ for $R = 2$ and some values of α. The corresponding eigenvalue for each α can be identified as the ϵ-coordinate of the point of intersection of the two curves. For the central Dirac-δ barrier case, $V_0 < 0$ [letting $V_0 = -g$ ($g > 0$)], the following energy equations can be derived: (i) $T(2\epsilon) = T(0) - Q\epsilon^{\alpha-1}$ and (ii) $T(0) - T(2\epsilon) + 2Q\epsilon^{\alpha-1} = \pm[9T^2(0) + 6T(2\epsilon)T(0) + T^2(2\epsilon) - 16T^2(\epsilon)]^{1/2}$, where $Q = 2\pi\hbar^\alpha D_\alpha/(a^{\alpha-1} g)$. The energy equations (i) and (ii) are plotted in the left and right panels of Fig. 2, respectively, for $Q = 2$.

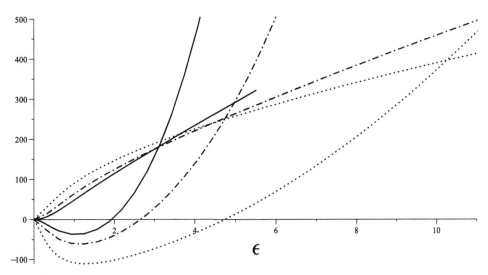

Fig. 1. Plots of the functions $f(\alpha, \epsilon)$ and $h(\alpha, \epsilon)$ for the case $V_0 > 0$ with $R = 2$ and $\alpha = 1.6$ (dotted curve), $\alpha = 1.8$ (dash-dotted curve), and $\alpha = 2.0$ (solid curve).

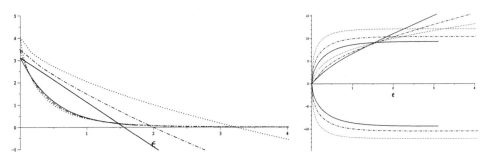

Fig. 2. Plots of the energy equations for the case $V_0 < 0$ with $Q = 2$ and $\alpha = 1.6$ (dotted curves), $\alpha = 1.8$ (dash-dotted curves), and $\alpha = 2.0$ (solid curves).

The wave function $\psi(x)$ can be obtained by inverse Fourier transforming $\tilde{\psi}(p)$. Furthermore, by a suitable choice of phase and application of Parseval's theorem,[3] $\int_{-\infty}^{\infty} \psi^*(x)\psi(x)dx = (2\pi\hbar)^{-1} \int_{-\infty}^{\infty} \tilde{\psi}^*(p)\tilde{\psi}(p)dp$, the normalized wave function for the case $V_0 > 0$ can be expressed as $\Psi(x) = N_\alpha[W\phi(x+a) - \phi(x) + Z\phi(x-a)]$, where $N_\alpha = \sqrt{\pi\lambda/\hbar}F(\alpha, W, Z)$ is the normalization constant, with $F(\alpha, W, Z) = [\alpha^{-2}(\alpha - 1)\pi(W^2 + Z^2 + 1)\csc(\pi/\alpha) - 4(W + Z)I(a\lambda/\hbar) + 2WZ\,I(2a\lambda/\hbar)]^{-1/2}$ from which we define $W = C_0(a)/2C_1(0)$, $Z = C_2(a)/2C_1(0)$, and $I(y) = \int_0^\infty \cos(yq)(q^\alpha + 1)^{-2}dq$ ($q = p/\lambda$), and the ϕ's are expressed in terms of Fox's H-function:[5]

$$\phi(y) = H_{2,3}^{2,1}\left[(\lambda/\hbar)^\alpha|y|^\alpha \left| \begin{matrix} (1-1/\alpha,1),(1/2,\alpha/2) \\ (0,\alpha),(1-1/\alpha,1),(1/2,\alpha/2) \end{matrix} \right. \right]. \tag{5}$$

Figure 3 plots this bound-state wave function for $W = Z$.

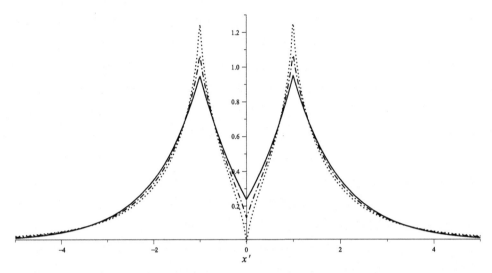

Fig. 3. Plot of the wave function Ψ/N_α as a function of $x' = x\lambda/\hbar$ for $\alpha = 1.6$ (dotted curve), $\alpha = 1.8$ (dash-dotted curve), and $\alpha = 2.0$ (solid curve) with $W = Z = 2$.

Case II: $E > 0$. For this case we let $\lambda^\alpha = E/D_\alpha$ ($\lambda > 0$). Using the property $f(x)\delta(x) = f(0)\delta(x)$ of the delta function (see also Ref. 3 for the treatment of single and double delta potentials for the case $E > 0$ using this property), we write $\tilde\psi(p)$ as
$$\tilde\psi(p) = A_1\delta(p-\lambda) + A_2\delta(p+\lambda) - \gamma_\alpha(|p|^\alpha - \lambda^\alpha)^{-1}[e^{iap/\hbar}C_0(a) - 2C_1(0) + e^{-iap/\hbar}C_2(a)].$$
Using this to find C_0, C_1, C_2 we obtain

$$UC_0(a) = \frac{\mu(2\rho l_1 - 3l_2^2 + 1)}{1 - l_2}M_0(a\lambda/\hbar) + 2\mu\rho M_1(0) + \frac{2\mu(l_2 - \rho l_1)}{1 - l_2}M_2(a\lambda/\hbar), \quad (6)$$

$$UC_1(0) = -\mu\rho M_0(a\lambda/\hbar) + \nu(1 + l_2)M_1(0) - \mu\rho M_2(a\lambda/\hbar), \quad (7)$$

$$UC_2(a) = \frac{2\mu(l_2 - \rho l_1)}{1 - l_2}M_0(a\lambda/\hbar) + \mu\rho M_1(0) + \frac{2\mu(2\rho l_1 + 1)}{1 - l_2}M_2(a\lambda/\hbar), \quad (8)$$

where we denote $\mu = [1 + \Lambda_\alpha^{-1}S(0)]^{-1}$, $\nu = [1 - 2\Lambda_\alpha^{-1}S(0)]^{-1}$, $\rho = \Lambda_\alpha^{-1}\nu S(a\lambda/\hbar)$, $l_j = \Lambda_\alpha^{-1}\mu S(ja\lambda/\hbar)$ ($j = 1, 2$), $U = 4\rho l_1 + l_2 + 1$, $M_0(a\lambda/\hbar) = M_2(-a\lambda/\hbar) = A_1 e^{-ia\lambda/\hbar} + A_2 e^{ia\lambda/\hbar}$, $M_1(0) = A_1 + A_2$, and $S(y) = 2\int_0^\infty \cos(yq)(q^\alpha - 1)^{-1}dq$ ($q = p/\lambda$); note from these definitions that $\nu l_1 = \mu\rho$.

The wave function $\psi(x)$ after inverse Fourier transforming $\tilde\psi(p)$ is $\psi(x) = A_1' e^{i\lambda x/\hbar} + A_2' e^{-i\lambda x/\hbar} + (2\hbar\Lambda_\alpha)^{-1}[C_0(a)\zeta(x+a) - 2C_1(0)\zeta(x) + C_2(a)\zeta(x-a)]$, where $A_j' = A_j/2\pi\hbar$ ($j = 1, 2$), the C_n's are those enumerated in Eqs. (6)–(8), and the ζ's are the following Fox's H-functions:

$$\zeta(y) = H_{2,3}^{2,1}\left[(\lambda/\hbar)^\alpha|y|^\alpha\,\middle|\,\begin{matrix}(1-1/\alpha,1),(1-[2+\alpha]/2\alpha,[2+\alpha]/2)\\(0,\alpha),(1-1/\alpha,1),(1-[2+\alpha]/2\alpha,[2+\alpha]/2)\end{matrix}\right]$$

$$-H_{2,3}^{2,1}\left[(\lambda/\hbar)^\alpha|y|^\alpha\,\middle|\,\begin{matrix}(1-1/\alpha,1),(1-[2-\alpha]/2\alpha,[2-\alpha]/2)\\(0,\alpha),(1-1/\alpha,1),(1-[2-\alpha]/2\alpha,[2-\alpha]/2)\end{matrix}\right]. \tag{9}$$

Acknowledgments

We are grateful to Dr. C. Bernido and Dr. M. V. Carpio-Bernido for their hospitality during our stay in Jagna for the workshop.

References

1. N. Laskin, Fractional quantum mechanics, *Phys. Rev. E* **63**, 3135 (2000).
2. N. Laskin, Fractional Schrödinger equation, *Phys. Rev. E* **66**, 056108 (2002).
3. E. C. de Oliveira, F. S. Costa, and J. Vaz, Jr., The fractional Schrödinger equation for delta potentials, *J. Math. Phys.* **51**, 123517 (2010).
4. S. H. Patil, Quadrupolar, triple δ-function potential in one dimension, *Eur. J. Phys.* **30**, 629 (2009).
5. A. M. Mathai, R. K. Saxena, and H. J. Haubold, *The H-Function: Theory and Applications* (Springer, New York, 2009).

7th Jagna International Workshop (2014)
International Journal of Modern Physics: Conference Series
Vol. 36 (2015) 1560015 (5 pages)
© The Authors
DOI: 10.1142/S2010194515600150

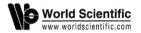

Lévy path integral approach to the fractional Schrödinger equation with delta-perturbed infinite square well

M. M. I. Nayga* and J. P. H. Esguerra

*National Institute of Physics, University of the Philippines-Diliman,
Quezon City 1101, Philippines*
mnayga@nip.upd.edu.ph

Published 2 January 2015

Using a path integral approach, we consider a fractional Schrödinger equation with delta-perturbed infinite square well. The Lévy path integral, which is generalized from the Feynman path intergal for the propagator, is expanded into a perturbation series. From this, the energy-dependent Green's function is obtained.

Keywords: Fractional quantum mechanics; path integral.

PACS Number: 03.65.Db

1. Introduction

Fractional quantum mechanics was first introduced by Laskin. It is described by the space-fractional Schrödinger equation (SFSE) containing the Riesz fractional operator. Following Feynman's path integral approach to quantum mechanics, Laskin generalized the path integral over Brownian motions to Lévy flights and obtained the space-fractional Schrödinger equation.[1,2]

Solutions to the space-fractional Schrödinger equation with linear potential, delta potential, infinite square well, and Coulumb potential, have already been obtained via piece-wise solution approach, momentum representation method, and, indirectly, the Lévy path integral approach.[3–5] However, despite the numerous works on fractional quantum mechanics, perturbation has not yet been explored. In this paper, we consider the space-fractional Schrödinger equation with perturbative terms using the Lévy path integral approach. We follow Grosche's perturbation expansion scheme[6,7] and obtained an energy-dependent Green's function for delta perturbations. As an example, we consider an infinite square well with delta-function perturbation.

2. Lévy path integral and fractional Schrödinger equation

If a particle starts from a point x_i at an initial time t_i and goes to a final point x_f at time t_f, its path $x(t)$ will have the property, $x(t_i) = x_i$ and $x(t_f) = x_f$. To get from the initial point to the final point, we define a propagator, $K_L(x_f, x_i; t_f - t_i)$, which is the sum over all of the paths that go between points (x_i, t_i) and (x_f, t_f). If a particle moves in a potential, then the propagator is written as

$$K_L(x_f, x_i; t_f - t_i) = \int_{x(t_i)=x_i}^{x(t_f)=x_f} Dx(t') \exp\left[-\frac{i}{\hbar} \int_{t_i}^{t_f} dt' V(x(t')) \right], \quad (1)$$

where $V(x(t'))$ is the potential energy as a functional of the Lévy particle path and the fractional path integral measure is defined as[2]

$$\int_{x(t_i)=x_i}^{x(t_f)=x_f} Dx(t') = \lim_{N \to \infty} \int dx_1...dx_{N-1} \left(\frac{iD_\alpha\epsilon}{\hbar}\right)^{-N/\alpha}$$

$$\times \prod_{j=1}^{N} L_\alpha\left[\left(\frac{\hbar}{iD_\alpha\epsilon}\right)^{1/\alpha} |x_j - x_{j-1}|\right]..., \quad (2)$$

where D_α is the generalized 'fractional diffusion coefficient' (has physical dimension, $[D_\alpha] = erg^{1-\alpha}cm^\alpha s^\alpha$, $D_\alpha = 1/2m$ for $\alpha = 2$, m denotes the mass of the particle), $x_0 = x_i$, $x_N = x_f$, $\epsilon = (t_f - t_i)/N$, and $L_\alpha(x)$ is the Lévy probability distribution function. For $\alpha = 2$, equation (2) is transformed to the Feynman free particle propagator.[2]

The propagator describes the evolution of the fractional quantum mechanical system in the following way,

$$\psi_f(x_f, t_f) = \int_{-\infty}^{+\infty} dx_i K_L(x_f, x_i; t_f - t_i)\psi_i(x_i, t_i), \quad (3)$$

where $\psi_i(x_i, t_i)$ is the fractional wave function of the initial state and $\psi_f(x_f, t_f)$ is the fractional wave function of the final state. Laskin derived the one-dimensional fractional Schrödinger equation as follows

$$i\hbar\frac{\partial\psi(x,t)}{\partial t} = [-D_\alpha(\hbar\nabla)^\alpha + V(x,t)]\psi(x,t), \quad (4)$$

where $(\hbar\nabla)^\alpha$ is the Riesz fractional derivative operator,

$$(\hbar\nabla)^\alpha\psi(x,t) = -\frac{1}{2\pi\hbar} \int_{-\infty}^{+\infty} dp e^{ipx/\hbar}|p|^\alpha \int_{-\infty}^{+\infty} e^{-ipx/\hbar}\psi(x,t)dx. \quad (5)$$

3. Path integration via summation of perturbation expansions

We follow Grosche's method for the time-ordered perturbation expansion.[6,7] We assume that we have a potential $W(x) = V(x) + \tilde{V}(x)$. The propagator corresponding to $V(x)$ is assumed to be known. We expand the propagator containing $\tilde{V}(x)$ in a perturbation expansion about $V(x)$ in the following way. The initial kernel corresponding to $V(x)$ propagates in Δt time unperturbed, then interacts with $\tilde{V}(x)$, propagates again in another Δt time unperturbed, and so on, up to the final state. We obtain the following expansion[6, 7]

$$K_L(x_f, x_i; t_f - t_i) = \int_{x(t_i)=x_i}^{x(t_f)=x_f} Dx(t') \exp\left[-\frac{i}{\hbar} \int_{t_i}^{t_f} dt'(V(x(t')) + \tilde{V}(x(t'))) \right]$$

$$= \int_{x(t_i)=x_i}^{x(t_f)=x_f} Dx(t') \exp\left[-\frac{i}{\hbar} \int_{t_i}^{t_f} dt' V(x(t')) \right]$$

$$+ \sum_{n=1}^{\infty} \left(\frac{-i}{\hbar} \right)^n \frac{1}{n!} \int_{x(t_i)=x_i}^{x(t_f)=x_f} Dx(t') \exp\left[-\frac{i}{\hbar} \int_{t_i}^{t_f} dt' V(x(t')) \right]$$

$$\times \left[\int_{t_i}^{t_f} dt' \, \tilde{V}(x(t')) \right]^n. \tag{6}$$

Introducing a time-ordering operator, the expansion becomes

$$K_L(x_f, x_i; t_f - t_i) = K_L^{(V)}(x_f, x_i; t_f - t_i) + \sum_{n=1}^{\infty} \left(\frac{-i}{\hbar} \right)^n \left[\prod_{k=1}^{n} \int_{t_i}^{t_k} dt_k \int_{-\infty}^{+\infty} dx_k \right]$$

$$\times K_L^{(V)}(x_1, x_i; t_1 - t_i) \, \tilde{V}(x_1)...K_L^{(V)}(x_n, x_{n-1}; t_n - t_{n-1})$$

$$\times \tilde{V}(x_n) K_L^{(V)}(x_f, x_n; t_f - t_n)$$

where $K_L^{(V)}$ is the fractional propagator for the unperturbed potential and again, it is assumed to be known. We have ordered time as $t_i < t_1 < t_2 < ... < t_f$ and paid attention to the fact that $K_L(t_k - t_{k-1})$ is different from zero only if $t_k > t_{k-1}$.

Now for an arbitrary potential $V(x)$ with an additional δ-perturbation, $W(x) = V(x) - \gamma\delta(x - a)$, the path integral is given by

$$K_L^{(\delta)}(x_f, x_i; t_f - t_i) = K_L^{(V)}(x_f, x_i; t_f - t_i) + \sum_{n=1}^{\infty} \left(\frac{-i\gamma}{\hbar} \right)^n \int_{t_i}^{t_f} dt_n...$$

$$\times \int_{t_i}^{t_1} dt_1 K_L^{(V)}(a, x_i; t_1 - t_i)...$$

$$\times K_L^{(V)}(a, a; t_n - t_{n-1}) K_L^{(V)}(x_f, a; t_f - t_n). \tag{7}$$

The energy-dependent Green's function for the unperturbed system is given by

$$G^{(V)}(x_f, x_i; E) = \frac{i}{\hbar} \int_0^{\infty} dT e^{iET/\hbar} K_L^{(V)}(x_f, x_i; t_f - t_i), T = t_f - t_i. \tag{8}$$

We also introduce the Green's function, $G^{(\delta)}(x_f, x_i; E)$ for the perturbed system in a similar manner as equation (8). The emerging geometric power series can be summed up due to the convolution theorem of the Fourier transformation, hence we have[6,7]

$$G^{(\delta)}(x_f, x_i; E) = G^{(V)}(x_f, x_i; E) - \frac{G^{(V)}(x_f, a; E)G^{(V)}(a, x_i; E)}{G^{(V)}(a, a; E) - 1/\gamma},$$ (9)

where it is assumed that $G^{(V)}(a, a; E)$ actually exists. The energy levels E_n of the perturbed system can be determined in a unique way by the denominator of $G^{(\delta)}(x_f, x_i; E)$.

4. The infinite square well with delta-perturbation

We first consider a particle in a potential $V(x)$ defined as

$$V(x) = \begin{cases} 0, & |x| \leq l \\ \infty, & |x| > l. \end{cases}$$ (10)

The fractional quantum-mechanical propagator for this system was already obtained by Dong,[4]

$$K_L^{(V)}(x_f, x_i; t_f - t_i) = \frac{1}{l}\sum_{n=1}^{\infty} \exp[-iE_n(t_f - t_i)/\hbar]\sin[k_n(x_i - l)]\sin[k_n(x_f - l)],$$

where

$$k_n = \frac{n\pi}{2l}, \quad E_n = D_\alpha \hbar^\alpha |k_n|^\alpha.$$ (11)

Solving the energy-dependent Green's function for this propagator yields

$$G^{(V)}(x_f, x_i; E) = \frac{1}{l}\sum_{n=1}^{\infty}\left(\frac{1}{E_n - E}\right)\sin[k_n(x_i - l)]\sin[k_n(x_f - l)].$$ (12)

Hence, from equation (9), the Green's function for the perturbed system is given by

$$G^{(\delta)}(x_f, x_i; E) = \frac{1}{l}\sum_{n=1}^{\infty}\left(\frac{1}{E_n - E}\right)\sin[k_n(x_i - l)]\sin[k_n(x_f - l)]$$

$$- \frac{1}{l^2}\sum_{n=1}^{\infty}\sum_{m=1}^{\infty}\left(\frac{1}{E_n - E}\right)\left(\frac{1}{E_m - E}\right)\sin[k_n(a - l)]\sin[k_n(x_f - l)]$$

$$\times \sin[k_m(x_i - l)]\sin[k_m(a - l)]$$

$$\times \left[\frac{1}{l}\sum_{n=1}^{\infty}\left(\frac{1}{E_n - E}\right)\sin^2[k_n(a - l)] - 1/\gamma\right]^{-1}.$$

5. Conclusion

We have expanded the Lévy path integral for the fractional quantum propagator in a perturabation series. An analogous expansion with the Feynman path integral was obtained. From the expanded propagator, the energy dependent Green's function for the delta-perturbed infinite square well was also obtained.

References

1. N. Laskin, "Fractional quantum mechanics," *Phys. lett. A 268*, pp. 268–305, 2000.
2. N. Laskin, "Fractional quantum mechanics and Lévy path integrals," *Phys. Rev. E 62*, pp. 3135–3145, 2000.
3. J. Dong and M. Xu, "Some solutions to the space fractional Schrödinger equation using momentum representation method," *J. Math. Phys. 48*, 072105 , 2007.
4. J. Dong, "Lévy path integral approach to the solution of the fractional Schrödinger equation with infinite square well," *arXiv:1301.3009v1 [math-ph]*, 2013.
5. E. C. de Oliveira, F. S. Costa, and J. Vaz Jr., "The fractional Schrödinger equation for delta potentials," *J. Math. Phys. 51*, 123517 , 2010.
6. C. Grosche, "Path integrals for potential problems wth δ-function perturbation," *J. Phys. A 23*, 5205, 1990.
7. C. Grosche, "Path integraton via summation of perturbation expansions and applications to totally reflecting boundaries and potential steps," *Phys. Rev. Lett. 71 (1)*, pp. 1–4, 1993.

7th Jagna International Workshop (2014)
International Journal of Modern Physics: Conference Series
Vol. 36 (2015) 1560016 (7 pages)
© The Authors
DOI: 10.1142/S2010194515600162

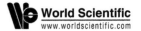

Fractional Brownian motion and polymers:
Learning from each other

J. Bornales

Physics Department, Mindanao State University-Iligan Institute of Technology,
Iligan City, 9200 Philippines
jinky.bornales@g.msuiit.edu.ph

L. Streit

Forschungszentrum BiBoS, Bielefeld University, D 33501 Bielefeld, Germany,
and
CCM, University of Madeira, P 9000-390 Funchal, Portugal
streit@physik.uni-bielefeld.de

Published 2 January 2015

Self-avoiding or self-repelling random paths, with motivation from their use in polymer physics, have been widely studied using the tools of mathematics, physics, and computer simulations. We illustrate this by three recent examples.

1. Introduction

Self-avoiding or self-repelling random path models for polymer configurations have been studied extensively in mathematics using combinatorics, stochastic analysis, in statistical mechanics, and in computer physics using Monte Carlo methods. Classical texts are e.g.[4] and[12], a recent review can be found in[17]. The field is highly interdisciplinary: the motivation came from chemistry, while physics provides structural intuition and far-reaching predictions, and computer simulations can check them out. The mathematical results are less far-reaching but provide the higher reliability characteristic of the mathematical approach; much remains to be done in the stochastic analysis setting.

Apart from self-avoiding random walks, a prominent realization is the Edwards model of self-repelling (or "weakly self-avoiding") Brownian paths, an example of models where self-crossings are not strictly forbidden but where there is an exponential penalty on self-crossings.[8]

Recently the Edwards model has been extended to fractional Brownian motion (fBm),[13] allowing for models of stiffer or curlier polymers than those described by classical Brownian motion.

It is in this context that we shall present report on progress on three fronts, where methods from stochastic analysis, arguments from statistical physics, and numerical computation have been employed.

2. Recent developments

2.1. *Varadhan's existence proof*

In the Edwards model self-repelling paths are described via a "Boltzmann factor" to suppress self-intersections of Brownian motion B :

$$G = \frac{1}{Z} \exp\left(-g \int_0^N ds \int_0^N dt \delta\left(B(s) - B(t)\right)\right)$$

with

$$Z = E\left(\exp\left(-g \int_0^N ds \int_0^N dt \delta\left(B(s) - B(t)\right)\right)\right).$$

The mathematical problem here lies with the existence of this exponential, how to make sense of

$$L = \int_0^N ds \int_0^N dt \delta\left(B(s) - B(t)\right)$$

One uses delta sequences to approximate the Dirac distribution

$$\delta_\varepsilon(x) := \frac{1}{(2\pi\varepsilon)^{d/2}} e^{-\frac{|x|^2}{2\varepsilon}}, \quad \varepsilon > 0,$$

$$L_\varepsilon := \int_0^l dt \int_0^t ds \, \delta_\varepsilon(B(t) - B(s)). \tag{1}$$

Removing the regularization depends on the dimension of the Brownian paths, it is straightforward for $d = 1$ but for $d \geq 2$ the expectation diverges

$$\lim_{\varepsilon \searrow 0} \mathbb{E}(L_\varepsilon) = \infty.$$

In $d = 2$ one needs to subtract the expectation, setting

$$L_\varepsilon^c = L_\varepsilon - \mathbb{E}(L_\varepsilon),$$

and will define the centered self-intersection local time as

$$L^c = \lim_{\varepsilon \searrow 0} L_\varepsilon^c.$$

In $d = 3$ a further, multiplicative renormalization is required,[20] but for $d = 2$ one is thus led to consider

$$\exp\left(-gL^c\right).$$

However, after centering L^c is unbounded below, and

$$\exp\left(-gL^c\right) \to \infty \text{ when } L^c \to -\infty.$$

So one needs to show that large values occur only with small probability such that the expectation is nevertheless finite. Varadhan[19] shows that

$$\mathbb{E}\left(\exp(-gL^c)\right) < \infty$$

and a bona fide probability distribution for planar self-repelling Brownian paths exists if $g > 0$ is sufficiently small. By a further scaling argument this existence result can be extended to all $g > 0$.

Varadhan's famous proof is based on a clever use of the Chebyshev inequality, using the logarithmic divergence of the expectation and an estimate of the rate of convergence

$$\|L^c - L_\varepsilon^c\|^2_{L^2(\mu)} \leq const.\varepsilon^a \text{ for all } a < 1/2.$$

Concerning this rate of convergence, in his words, "*...this is the most difficult step of all and requires considerable estimation*". Hence an alternate proof may be of interest.

Using the tools of White Noise Analysis, in the particular multiple Wiener integral or "chaos" decomposition of the self-intersection local time[9] it is straightforward to show[2]

Theorem 2.1. *Let $T > 0$ be given. Then*

$$\|L_\varepsilon^c(T) - L^c(T)\|^2 \leq C\varepsilon^\alpha \; \forall \alpha < 1.$$

Apart from a simplified proof one notes the doubling of the convergence rate α.

Remark 2.1. While a generalisation of the Varadhan existence proof to fBm is now available,[13] its extension to arbitrary coupling constants g remains an open challenge.

2.2. *The Flory index*

Contrary to the above, the scaling behavior of self-repelling paths is not (yet) accessible to strict mathematical arguments, with the exception of the unphysical one-dimensional case.[14]

The question, in physical terms, is about the "end-to-end-length" R of polymer, and how it grows as one increases the number N of monomers in the chain. Mathematically, for a (fractional) Brownian path $x = B^H$, one has

$$\mathbb{E}\left(x(N) - x(0)^2\right) = N^{2\nu}$$

with ν equal to the "Hurst index" H which characterizes the fBm. The suppression of self-intersections, "excluded volume effect" in physics terminology, will make the paths swell and one expects $\nu > H$.

Flory's famous formula[10]

$$\nu = \frac{3}{d+2}$$

for spatial dimensions $d = 1, 2, 3$ was based on a flawed mean field argument[12] but is remarkably accurate.[17] Recently it was extended to the fractional case,[1] with

$$\nu_H = \frac{2H+2}{d+2}.$$

Computer simulations appear to support this formula at least for $d = 1$. In Refs. [5] and[6] the original self-avoiding Brownian model has been extended to the case where k-fold intersections are tolerated, and only higher order ones penalized. Informally this would correspond to the use of higher order self-intersection local times

$$L^{(k)}(N) \equiv \int_0^N dt \int_0^N d^k s \prod_{l=1}^k \delta \left(x(t) - x(s_l) \right).$$

For a rigorous mathematical discussion of such higher order intersection local times and the necessary renormalizations to make them well-defined see e.g.[7].

Putting aside the problems of a rigorous definition, one can invoke, simple, dimensional arguments would lead to

$$\nu_{H,k}(d) = \frac{2H+k+1}{kd+2} \tag{2}$$

which now covers all values of the dimension d, the Hurst index H, and the tolerance level k, up to the limiting dimensions where there are no more self-intersections, see formula (3) below.

The singularity of higher order self-intersection local times and the non-Markovian nature of fBm complicate the mathematical analysis of scaling even beyond the classical Brownian case. In this light it is remarkable that for

$$Hd = \frac{k+1}{k}$$

the formula (2) produces

$$\nu_{H,k}(d) = H \tag{3}$$

i.e. there is no swelling from the suppression of self-intersections. This coincides in fact with a rigorous mathematical result: Talagrand[18] proves that indeed with probability 1 fBm has no $(k+1)$-tuple points whenever

$$Hd \geq \frac{k+1}{k}.$$

On the other hand one notes that for $d = 1$ the formula (2) would predict increased swelling for $k > 1$; also in the Bm case one expects Wilson type renormalization to induce a $k = 1$ term in the renormalized interaction,[16] hence the usual Flory scaling also for k-tolerant models.

2.3. *Computational results*

In view of the difficulties confronting a mathematical investigation computer simulations suggest themselves.

Results in this direction are based on a discretized version of the k-tolerant model, with monomer positions

$$x_k = B^H(k), k = 0, 1, 2, ..., N - 1.$$

As for the self-intersection local time $L^{(k)}$, one notes that, informally, we can express it in terms of the local time $L(N, u)$, given informally by

$$L(N, u) = \int_0^N dt \delta \left(x(t) - u \right).$$

Indeed one has

$$L^{(k)}(N) = \int_0^N dt \int_0^N d^k s \prod_{l=1}^k \delta \left(x(t) - x(s_l) \right)$$

$$= \int_0^N du \left(\int_0^N dt \delta \left(x(t) - u \right) \right)^{k+1}$$

$$= \int_0^N du L^{k+1}(N, u)$$

and the latter is straightforward to discretize. Monte Carlo computations with importance sampling[15] are then based on a conformation energy

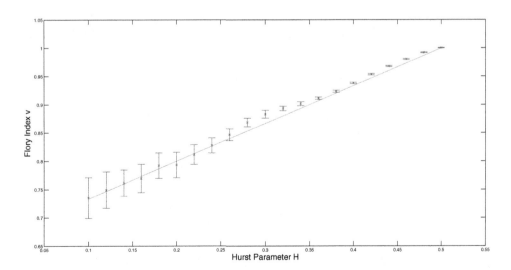

Fig. 1.

$$E(x) = E_0(x) + gE_1(x)$$

where E_0 is obtained by inverting the fBm covariance matrix, and the excluded volume energy is given by a discretized version of $L^{(k)}$.

Preliminary results for $d = 1$, $k = 1$, and $0 < H < 1/2$ give encouraging results, see Fig. 1. The straight line corresponds to formula (2) for $k = 1$; extensive precision calculations are under way[3].

Acknowledgments

This work was financed by Portuguese national funds through FCT - Fundação para a Ciência e Tecnologia within the project PTDC/MAT-STA/1284/2012.

References

1. J. Bornales, M.J. Oliveira, L. Streit: Self-repelling fractional Brownian motion — a generalized Edwards model for chain polymers. In L. Accardi, W. Freudenberg, M. Ohya (Eds.), Q. Probability and WNA 30, 389–401. World Scientific Singapore, 2013.
2. W. Bock, M.J. Oliveira, J.L. Silva, L.Streit: Polymer Measure: Varadhan's Renormalization Revisited, preprint, 2014. arXiv:1405.7150 [math-ph]
3. W. Bock, J. Bornales, S. Eleuterio (to be published).
4. J. des Cloiseaux and G. Jannik, Polymers in Solutions: Their Modelling and Structure. Oxford University Press 1990.
5. R. Dekeyzer, A. Maritan, A. Stella, Excluded-volume effects in linear polymers: Universality of generalized self-avoiding walks. Phys. Rev. B 31, 4659–4662 (1985).
6. R. Dekeyzer, A. Maritan, A. Stella, Random walks with intersections: Static and dynamic fractal properties. Phys. Rev. A 36, 2338–2351 (1987).
7. S. Mendonça, L. Streit: Multiple Intersection Local Times in Terms of White Noise. IDAQP 4, 533 (2001).
8. S. F. Edwards, The statistical mechanics of polymers with excluded volume. Proc. Roy. Soc. 85, 613-624 (1965).
9. M. Faria, T. Hida, L. Streit, H. Watanabe: Intersection Local Times as Generalized White Noise Functional. Acta Appl. Math. **46**, 351 (1997).
10. P.J. Flory, Principles of Polymer Chemistry. Cornell University Press. 1953
11. M.E. Fisher, J. Phys. Soc. Japan 26 Suppl. 44 (1969)
12. P. G. de Gennes, Scaling Concepts in Polymer Physics. Cornell Univ. Press, Ithaca, NY. (1979)
13. M. Grothaus, M.J. Oliveira, J.-L. Silva, L. Streit: Self-avoiding fBm - The Edwards model. J. Stat. Phys. 145, 1513–1523 (2011).
14. R. van der Hofstad, W. König, A Survey of One-Dimensional Random Polymers. J. Stat. Physics, **103**, 915–944 (2001).
15. N. Metropolis, A.W. Rosenbluth, M.N. Rosenbluth, A.H. Teller, and E. Teller: Equation of State Calculations by Fast Computing Machines. Journal of Chemical Physics 21, 1087–1092 (1953).
16. Y. Oono, K. Freed: Conformation Space Renormalizationof Polymers I. J. Chem. Phys. 75, 993–1008 (1981).
17. A. Pelissetto, E. Vicari: Critical phenomena and renormalization-group theory. Phys. Reports **368**, 549–727 (2002).
18. M. Talagrand: Multiple points of trajectories of multiparameter fractional Brownian motion. *Probab. Theory Related Fields* **112**, 545–563 (1998).

19. S. R. S. Varadhan: Appendix to *"Euclidean quantum field theory"* by K. Symanzik, in: R. Jost, ed., Local Quantum Theory, Academic Press, New York, p. 285 (1970)

20. M. J. Westwater: On Edwards' model for long polymer chains. Comm. Math. Phys.72, 103–205 (1980).

7th Jagna International Workshop (2014)
International Journal of Modern Physics: Conference Series
Vol. 36 (2015) 1560017 (7 pages)
© The Authors
DOI: 10.1142/S2010194515600174

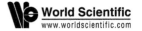

Fractional Brownian modeled linear polymer chains with one dimensional Metropolis Monte Carlo simulation

J. P. B. Sambo*, B. V. Gemao and J. B. Bornales

*Department of Physics, College of Science and Mathematics,
Mindanao Sate University - Iligan Institute of Technology,
Iligan City, 9200, Philippines*
*japhisam@gmail.com

Published 2 January 2015

The scaling expression for fractional Brownian modeled linear polymer chains was obtained both theoretically and numerically. Through the probability distribution of fractional Brownian paths, the scaling was found out to be $\langle R^2 \rangle \sim N^{2H}$, where R is the end-to-end distance of the polymer chain, N is the number of monomer units and H is the Hurst parameter. Numerical data was generated through the use of Monte Carlo simulation implementing the Metropolis algorithm. Results show good agreement between numerical and theoretical scaling constants after some parameter optimization. The probability distribution confirmed the Gaussian nature of fractional Brownian motion and the behavior is not affected by varying values of the Hurst parameter and of the number of monomer units.

Keywords: Polymer; fracional Brownian; Monte Carlo; scaling.

1. Introduction

Many polymer models have been established in order to describe polymer systems accurately. One of the most commonly used is the Brownian model or the freely-jointed chain model where the polymer chain is seen as a series of statistically independent and identical segments connected to each other, forming a linear chain[1]. This type of polymer chain can be described as a simple random walk. For more realistic chains, the excluded volume effect may be added to the system in order to avoid self-crossings as seen in models such as the Edwards and the Domb-Joyce models[2,3].

To describe linear polymer chains, the end-to-end vector, R, is used and the scaling expression for the system is established in order to relate the end-to-end vector, R, to the number of monomer units in polymer chain, N[4]. This expression takes the form $R \sim N^{\upsilon_H}$, where υ_H is the scaling constant. For the Brownian case in real polymer chains, the Flory index, given by $\upsilon_H = \frac{3}{d+2}$ where d is the dimension, is the established scaling constant[5]. However, the Brownian model is fit only for good solvents and is not appropriate for poor solvents and long-range repulsion solvents[4].

The fractional Brownian motion has been suggested for polymer models as it is a more general entity in which Brownian motion is a special case. It has been recently studied by Bornales et al. but the model includes the excluded volume effect which is fit for real chains[6]. Results from the study showed that the scaling constant is dependent on a variable parameter called the Hurst parameter, H, which means that different scaling expressions can be derived from the general expression itself, thereby possibly catering to different polymer configurations and eventually to different solvent types.

In this paper, the scaling expression for purely fractional Brownian modeled linear polymer chains is obtained by two methods - first, by solving it analytically from the probability distribution of fractional Brownian paths; second, by implementing numerical methods using Metropolis algorithm Monte Carlo simulation.

2. The Scaling Expression for Fractional Brownian motion

2.1. *Properties of fractional Brownian motion*

As suggested in studies such as those of Bornales *et al.*, fractional Brownian motion is a more generalized approach than the pure Brownian motion by providing a general correlation expression between Brownian paths controlled by the variable H, called the Hurst parameter. Also, as shown in the study by Sarkar, the expectation value for the square of the distance between two fBm paths depends on the Hurst parameter. This means that for different values of the Hurst parameter, different values of R^2 arise, making the variable H a parameter that may describe polymer solvent type.

Fractional Brownian motion has three major properties:

It is a continuous Gaussian chain. Therefore, its probability distribution is similar to the form[1],

$$P(N, x) = \frac{1}{\sqrt{2\pi \langle x^2 \rangle}} exp\left(-\frac{x^2}{2 \langle x^2 \rangle}\right). \tag{1}$$

Fractional Brownian paths have stationary increments[7],

$$\left\langle \left(B_t^H - B_s^H\right)^2\right\rangle = E\left[\left(B_t^H - B_s^H\right)^2\right]$$
$$= |t - s|^{2H}. \tag{2}$$

From the expression given in Equation (2), the correlation between fBm paths[6]

$$E\left[\left(B_t^H B_s^H\right)^2\right] = \frac{1}{2}\left(t^{2H} + s^{2H} - |t - s|^{2H}\right). \tag{3}$$

where H is called the Hurst parameter which has values, $0 < H < 1$.

It is self similar. Consider B_t^H as a Brownian path, then self-similarity[8] is defined by

$$\frac{1}{a^H} B_{at}^H = b_t^H \tag{4}$$

for $t \geq 0$ and $a > 0$, where b_t^H is a random variable of the same probability distribution as B_{at}^H.

All of these properties make fractional Brownian motion a more general model since it is able to cater to chains that have monomer interactions within them. The Brownian case is obtained when $H = \frac{1}{2}$, where the value for the correlation between Brownian paths is zero.

2.2. Derivation for the scaling expression

The expectation value of the square of the end-to-end distance of a linear polymer chain in fractional Brownian model is given in terms of the probability distribution and the expression is given as[6]

$$\langle R^2 \rangle = Z \int_0^N x^2 exp \left(-\beta \frac{(x_t, H_0 x_s)}{2} \right) dx, \tag{5}$$

where x is a Brownian path and β and Z are constants and H_0 carries the correlation between monomer positions defined by the equation $E\left[(B_t^H \cdot B_s^H)^2\right]^{-1} = H_0$. It is possible to make use of changing the variables to eliminate the constant β from the exponential term. Letting $x = \beta^{-\frac{1}{2}} a$, then $x^2 = \beta^{-1} a^2$. Now, applying this change, the expression for $\langle R^2 \rangle$ becomes

$$\langle R^2 \rangle = Z \int_0^N a^2 exp \left(-\beta \frac{\left(\beta^{-\frac{1}{2}} a, H_0 \beta^{-\frac{1}{2}} a \right)}{2} \right) da. \tag{6}$$

Simplifying the inner product expression, we may express Equation (6) as

$$\langle R^2 \rangle = Z \int_0^N a^2 exp \left(-\frac{H_0 a^2}{2} \right) da. \tag{7}$$

Note that,

$$\langle x^2 \rangle \sim \int a^2 exp \left[-\frac{c^2}{2} x^2 \right] dx. \tag{8}$$

Implementing Equation (8) to the expression given in Equation (7), $\langle R^2 \rangle$ becomes

$$\langle R^2 \rangle \sim ZE\left[x^2\right] = ZE\left[\left(B_N^H\right)^2\right]. \tag{9}$$

Since fBm is self-similar, then $B_N^H = N^H b^H$. Applying this to Equation (9) gives

$$\langle R^2 \rangle \sim ZN^{2H} E\left[\left(b^H\right)^2\right]. \tag{10}$$

From Equation (10), the scaling expression for fractional Brownian Motion is derived

$$\langle R^2 \rangle \sim N^{2H}.$$ (11)

This result is similar to that shown in the study by Sarkar where the expectation value for R^2 is given by a general formula[8]

$$E\left[\left(B_t^H - B_s^H\right)^2\right] = c\left(H\right)\left|t - s\right|^{2H}.$$ (12)

3. Simulation Methods

This study makes use of the Metropolis Monte Carlo simulation methods to produce numerical results. In order to attain the closest approximation to the average end-to-end distance of the polymer chain, the simulation method makes use of random generation of polymer configurations. A polymer configuration of known energy is generated first, then it is updated through randomly changing the position of one monomer unit. Doing this causes a new polymer configuration, as shown in the Figure 1, and thus corresponding to a new energy value.

Since it is assumed that the expectation value R^2 is in equilibrium condition, it is also necessary to reach the lowest possible energy for the polymer configuration. To achieve this, the simulation method implements a filtering condition where the new energy value should be less than the previous energy or should be less than the random number from 0 to 1 in order to be accepted as the new polymer configuration. This process is iterated multiple times in order to make the closest approximation and reach the most stable energy. Simulation results give values for $\ln\left(\langle R^2 \rangle^{\frac{1}{2}}\right)$ with the corresponding $\ln(N)$ values. The scaling expression is obtained as follows

$$ln\left(\langle R^2 \rangle^{\frac{1}{2}}\right) \approx \upsilon_H ln\left(N\right)$$

$$\langle R^2 \rangle^{\frac{1}{2}} \approx N^{\upsilon_H}$$

$$\langle R^2 \rangle \approx N^{2\upsilon_H}.$$

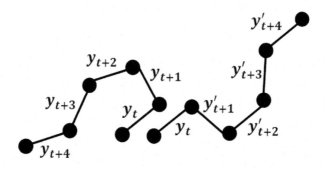

Fig. 1.   Changing one monomer unit in a linear chain.

Simulation codes were written by Dr. Wolfgang Bock of University of Kaiserslautern, Germany and Dr. Samuel Eleuterio of Unibersidade Tecnica de Lisboa, Portugal, along with their team in Germany, headed by Dr. Ludwig Streit, who are in collaborative work with the Physics Department, College of Science and Mathematics, Mindanao State University Iligan Institute of Technology, Iligan City, Philippines. The simulations were processed using C programming language.

4. Results and Discussion

Numerical data were obtained for Hurst parameter values of 0.1, 0.2, 0.3, 0.4, 0.5, 0.6, 0.7, 0.8 and 0.9. The number of monomer units was also varied from a range of 200 to 850 monomers with increments of 50. The results were plotted in a $\ln(N)$ vs $\ln\left(\langle R^2\rangle^{\frac{1}{2}}\right)$ where the slope was taken in order to find the scaling constant as shown in Figures 2, 3, 4 and 5.

From the plots illustrated, it can be inferred that as the value of H increases, the slope also increases but remains the same for $H \geq \frac{1}{2}$. Note that from the properties of fBm, for $H \leq \frac{1}{2}$, the fBm paths are negatively correlated and thus would correspond to an anti-persistent chain[8]. To better understand the results

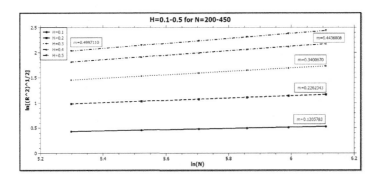

Fig. 2.   Plots for H-values of 0.1, 0.2, 0.3, 0.4, and 0.5, for $N = 200$–450 with slopes.

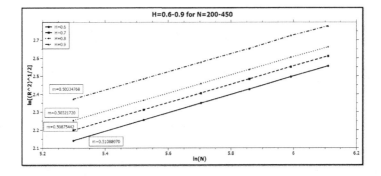

Fig. 3.   Plots for H-values of 0.6, 0.7, 0.8, and 0.9, for $N = 200$–450 with slopes.

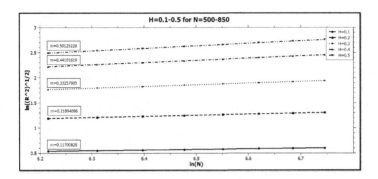

Fig. 4. Plots for H-values of 0.1, 0.2, 0.3, 0.4, and 0.5, for $N = 500$–850 with slopes.

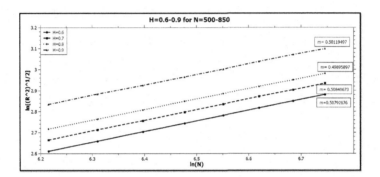

Fig. 5. Plots for H-values of 0.6, 0.7, 0.8, and 0.9, for $N = 500$–850 with slopes.

Table 1. Tabulated values for the simulated and the theoretical scaling constants for varying H, $r = 1$, $N = 200$–850.

(H)	Slope Obtained	
	$N = 200$–450	$N = 500$–850
0.1	0.1205783	0.11700828
0.2	0.2262343	0.21894096
0.3	0.340067	0.33257905
0.4	0.4436808	0.44101619
0.5	0.499711	0.50125228
0.6	0.51088970	0.50792676
0.7	0.50875442	0.50840673
0.8	0.50321720	0.49895897
0.9	0.50334768	0.50119497

obtained, the slope values are tabulated along with the corresponding H-value and the theoretical prediction. Note that the theoretical expression is given as $\langle R^2 \rangle \sim N^{2H}$, then the expected scaling constant is $\upsilon_H = H$.

Results show that the polymer configurations change with the various values of H for $H < 0.5$ and they follow the expected shrinking of the polymer chain, although exact values of the scaling constant give a slightly bigger deviation from the theoretical expectations. For the case of $H > 0.5$, the scaling constants remain to be the same as that of $H = 0.5$, which may be errors in the simulation process. The errors from the simulation results are yet to be investigated by varying some simulation parameters.

References

1. Rubinstein, M., and Colby, R.H., *Polymer Physics*. Oxford University Press (2003).
2. Edwards, S.F., *The statistical mechanics of polymers with excluded volume*. Proc. Phys. Sci. 85, **613-625** (1965).
3. Domb, C., and Joyce, G.S., *Cluster expansion for a polymer chain*. J. Physics C 5, **956-976** (1972).
4. de Gennes, P.G., *Scaling Concepts in Polymer Physics.*, Cornell University Press, Ithaca, New York, (1979).
5. Flory, P.J., *Principles of Polymer Chemistry*. Cornell University Press (1953).
6. Bornales, J., Oliveira, M., and Streit, L., *Self-Repelling Fractional Brownian Motion — A Generalized Edwards Model* arXiv:1106.377v2. (2011).
7. Hammond, A., Sheffield, S., *Power law Polya's urn and fractional Brownian motion*. Springer-Verlag, Berlin, (2012).
8. Sarkar, S., *Fractional Brownian Motion: Long range dependency, Markov property, Simulation strategy-A review*. Term Paper submitted for Stochastic Process Course in Spring, (2008).

7th Jagna International Workshop (2014)
International Journal of Modern Physics: Conference Series
Vol. 36 (2015) 1560018 (7 pages)
© The Authors
DOI: 10.1142/S2010194515600186

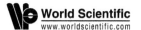

On the diffusion of alpha-helical proteins in solvents

Wilson I. Barredo

Department of Physics
Mindanao State University (MSU)-Iligan Institute of Technology
Iligan City, 9200, Philippines
Department of Physics, Mindanao State University
Marawi City, 9700, Philippines
barredo1234@yahoo.com

Jinky B. Bornales

Department of Physics
Mindanao State University (MSU)-Iligan Institute of Technology
Iligan City, 9200, Philippines
jbornales@gmail.com

Christopher C. Bernido

Research Center for Theoretical Physics
Central Visayan Institute Foundation
Jagna, Bohol, 6308, Philippines
cbernido@mozcom.com

Henry P. Aringa

Department of Physics, Mindanao State University
Marawi City, 9700, Philippines
henparinga@yahoo.com

Published 2 January 2015

The winding probability function for a biopolymer diffusing in a crowded cell is obtained with the drift coefficient $f(s)$ involving Bessel functions of general form $f(s) = kJ_{2p+1}(\nu s)$. The variable s is the length along the chain and ν is a constant which can be used to simulate the frequency of appearance of a certain type of amino acid. Application of a particular case $p = 3$ to protein chains is carried out for different alpha helical proteins found in the Protein Data Bank (PDB). Analysis of our results leads us to an empirical formula that can be used to conveniently predict k/D and ν, where D is the diffusion coefficient of various α-helical proteins in solvents.

Keywords: Diffusion coefficient; α-helical proteins; winding probability.

1. Introduction

In this paper, we show that from the results obtained earlier [1-3] for myoglobin and ferritin using the white noise functional approach in modeling the alpha-helical secondary structure of the protein, other α-helical proteins can also be simulated using Brownian paths. In particular, the Fokker-Plank equation is solved to obtain the probability density function from which winding probabilities $W(n, L)$ are calculated. The various helical protein conformations are then viewed as arrays of diffusion paths modulated by a drift coefficient involving Bessel functions of general order $f(s) = J_{2p+1}(\text{vs})$, in particular the case for $p = 3$. We then apply this to investigate the diffusion of proteins consisting mainly of α-helical conformations.

Development of reliable methods of predicting diffusion coefficients for proteins and other macromolecules is of interest since diffusion is involved in a number of biochemical processes such as protein aggregation, transport in intercellular media and the protein folding process [4]. Hence, how proteins diffuse inside the cell has been the subject of recent experimental and theoretical studies. Simple scaling and distribution relationships have been derived from recent databases to describe some of the physical properties of proteins in cellular proteomes [5]. The results show that many properties of proteins, including their sizes, stabilities, folding rates and diffusion coefficients depend simply on the chain length N. For instance, molecular dynamics simulations have been done to predict diffusion coefficients of four proteins: Cytochrome c (1HRC), lysozyme (1BWI), α-chymotrypsinogen-A (1EX3), and ovalbumin (1OVA) in aqueous solution. J. Wang and T. Hou [5] have also compared molecular diffusion coefficients with experimental values.

2. Modeling of the Polymer

In investigating helical structures of proteins, we use the circular cylindrical coordinates, $\mathbf{r} = (\rho, \theta, z)$, and take a winding polymer oriented along the z-axis. The polymer conformation can be viewed as random walk consisting of N steps which starts at point $\mathbf{r}_0$ and ends at some point $\mathbf{r}_1$. We can simplify the study of the winding behavior of a biopolymer by projecting the paths on the ρ–θ plane and consider a polymer chain which lies on the plane with endpoints at $\rho_0 = (\rho_0, \theta_0)$ and $\rho_1 = (\rho_1, \theta_1)$. However, for a typical α-helical conformation, the radius of a helix is known and, hence, we can fix the radial variable at $\rho = R$. From this scenario, a polymer which winds around the z-axis projects a circular structure on the ρ–θ plane. The probability density function can then be written as [3],

$$P(\theta_1, \theta_0; L) = \int exp\left\{ -\frac{1}{l} \int_0^L \left[R\frac{d\theta}{ds} - \frac{l}{2D}f(s) \right]^2 ds \right\} D[\theta]. \qquad (1)$$

Here, $L = Nl$ is the length of the polymer with l the length of each monomer, D is the diffusion constant and $f(s)$ the drift coefficient.

To reflect the varying interactions of the different amino acids in an aqueous environment, the value of the drift coefficient $f(s)$, with $0 \le s \le L$, can also vary at each length segment along the chainlike molecule. Corresponding to the path, θ can be parameterized as:

$$\theta(s) = \theta_0 + (\sqrt{l}/R)B(s) \tag{2}$$

where θ_0 is an initial value and B the Brownian fluctuation. Eq. (2) deals with paths confined to a circular topology. The paths can be classified topologically and characterized by winding numbers [6-11] $n = 0, \pm 1, \pm 2, \ldots$ where, $n > 0$ signifies n turns counterclockwise around the origin; $n < 0$ means $|n|$ turns clockwise, and $n = 0$ signifies no winding. With Eq. (2), an evaluation of Eq. (1) using white noise calculus yields the result [3],

$$P(\theta_1, \theta_0) = \sum_{n=-\infty}^{+\infty} P_n, \tag{3}$$

where,

$$P_n = \sqrt{\frac{R^2}{\pi l L}} \exp\left[-\frac{R^2}{lL}\left(\theta_0 - \theta_1 + 2\pi n + \frac{l}{2DR}\int_0^L f(s)\,ds\right)^2\right]. \tag{4}$$

Equation (4) is the probability function for an n-times winding of a path around the z-axis. The probability that a helical conformation has a polypeptide winding n-times about the z-axis is given by, $W(n, L) = P_n/P$. For an arbitrary initial point, we let $\theta_0 = \theta_1$, and we obtain [3],

$$W(n, L) = \sqrt{\frac{4\pi}{lL}} \frac{exp\left[-\frac{R^2}{lL}\left(2\pi n + \frac{l}{2DR}\int_0^L f(s)\,ds\right)^2\right]}{\boldsymbol{\theta_3}\left(\frac{1}{4DR}\right)\int_0^L f(s)\,ds}, \tag{5}$$

where $\boldsymbol{\theta_3}(u)$ is the theta function [12]. We note that Eq. (5) is an exact result obtained by evaluating Eq. (1). The interaction of each amino acid with the aqueous environment as well as with other monomers would be reflected in the drift coefficient $f(s)$, as s ranges from 0 to L along the length of a biopolymer. The $f(s)$ in turn serves as a modulating function affecting the winding probability $W(n, L)$ that describes a specific winding conformation. The particular drift coefficient used in this study is described in the next section.

3. Besselian Drift Coefficient of Order $2p + 1$

The drift coefficient, $f(s) = kJ_{2p+1}(\nu s)$, where $J_{2p+1}(\nu s)$ is a Bessel function, can be integrated over ds,

$$\int_0^L f(s)\,ds = (k/v)\left[1 - J_0(vL) - 2\sum_{m=1}^{p} J_{2m}(vL)\right], \tag{6}$$

with $p \geq 1$ [12]. Eq. (6) is then used in Eq. (5) to get the winding probability,

$$W(n, L) = R\sqrt{\frac{4\pi}{Ll}} \exp \times \left[\theta_3 \left(\frac{kl}{4DRv} \left[1 - J_0(vL) - 2\sum_{m=1}^{p} J_{2m}(vL)\right]\right)\right]^{-1}. \quad (7)$$

For long polymers $L = Nl >> 1$, $\boldsymbol{\theta_3}(u) \approx 1$, and the probability for a helical conformation with a winding number n becomes:

$$W(n, L) \approx R\sqrt{\frac{4\pi}{Ll}} \exp \left\{-\frac{R^2}{Ll} \left[2\pi n + \frac{kl}{2DRv}\right.\right.$$

$$\left.\left. \times \left(1 - J_0(vL) - 2\sum_{m=1}^{p} J_{2m}(vL)\right)\right]^2\right\}. \quad (8)$$

4. Application

We take the case $p = 3$ of the drift coefficient $f(s) = kJ_{2p+1}(vs) = kJ_7(vs)$ [1] and Eq. (6) reduces to:

$$\int f(s)ds = (k/v)\{1 - J_0(vL) - 2[J_2(vL) + J_4(vL) + J_6(vL)]\}. \quad (9)$$

The winding probability $W(n, L)$ is the same as Eq. (8), but with only $m = 1$, 2, 3 contributing to the summation term in the exponential. We use the general properties of proteins, $R = 0.25$ nm, $l = 0.15$ nm, and 3.6 residues per helical turn for different alpha helical proteins. The graphs of $W(n, L)$ versus length L are simulated in order to find the values of k/D and v that will mimic their experimentally verified features.

For example, myoglobin (4MBN) has only one chain with total length of 153 residues, with alpha helical segments about 80% of its length or about 123 residues, and with 11 helices based on PDB. Therefore this protein has about 123 residues divided by 3.6 residues/turns or about 34 helical turns and a length of $L = 0.15(153)$ nm ≈ 23 nm. Plotting the winding probability $W(-n, L)$ versus length L using the above data, the values of $v = 1.93$/nm and $k/D = 1420$/nm were found giving 11 peaks (Figure 1). The peaks apparently correspond to 11 helices of Myoglobin (4MBN), and the negative n signifies that this protein is right-handed.

The method above was used for other alpha-helical proteins presented in Table 1, with the values of k/D and v for each alpha-helical protein giving a good one-to-one correspondence between the number of peaks in the graph of $W(-n, L)$ versus length L and the number of helical segments based on data from PDB for each of the proteins.

One can observe in Table 1 that longer proteins have larger k/D values and shorter proteins have smaller values of k/D in aqueous solvent. These results agree with experimental observations [14]. In general, larger proteins diffuse slower and smaller ones diffuse faster in aqueous solvents. The results also agree with theoretical results based on the Stokes-Einstein theory [4]. The model therefore, has the

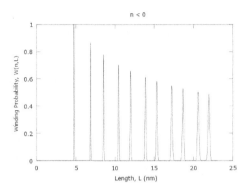

Fig. 1.   4MBN: Graph of $W(-n, L)$ versus length for $\nu = 1.93/\text{nm}$ and $k/D = 1420/\text{nm}$.

Table 1.   Properties of alpha helical proteins with the simulated values of k/D and ν.

Protein (PBD code)	Length (# of Residues)	% alpha (# of Residues)	# of helices	# of turns	ν (1/nm)	k/D (1/nm)
2K9J	42	57% (24)	1	7	1.30	490
3IA3-A[+]	91	71% (65)	3	18	1.30	490
2JUW	80	76% (61)	4	17	1.76	640
2I15	135	59% (80)	5	23	1.29	680
2HMZ	113	69% (79)	6	22	1.65	758
3IA3-D[++]	145	64% (93)	9	26	1.68	800
2MHB	141	73% (104)	9	29	1.79	1120
4MBN	153	80% (123)	11	34	1.93	1420
2O9D	234	71% (167)	12	47	1.36	1290
4E4V	485	63% (310)	31	86	1.48	2690
2YNS	490	64% (314)	33	87	1.53	2759
4BA3	496	64% (319)	34	89	1.55	2839

Note: [+]3IA3 chain A, [++]3IA3 chain D, and the rest of the above proteins are chain A if there are more than one chain.

potential for describing the general properties of a protein in aqueous solvent. The discouraging feature of this model, however, is that to obtain the values of k/D and ν for the number of peaks to correspond to the helices for each protein being investigated, one had to resort to trial and error scheme. In the graph of $W(-n, L)$ versus length, the desired number of peaks can only be obtained after adjusting several times the two parameters, ν and k/D. Therefore, an empirical formula has been developed to avoid this difficulty.

4.1. *Construction of an Empirical Formula*

In developing the empirical formula, the linear dependence of the values of k/D of the proteins presented in Table 1 to the number of helices was taken into account.

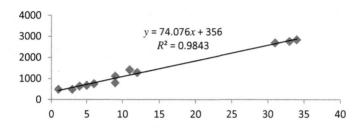

Fig. 2. Plot of k/D versus number of helices.

Table 2. Simulated values compared with predicted values of ν and k/D.

Protein (PBD code)	Length (# of Residues)	% alpha (# of Residues)	Simulated $\nu(1/nm)$	Simulated $k/D(1/nm)$	Predicted $\nu(1/nm)$	Predicted $k/D(1/nm)$
2K9J	42	57% (24)	1.30	490	1.49	395.67
3IA3-A+	91	71% (65)	1.30	490	1.415	612.92
2JUW	80	76% (61)	1.76	640	1.83	724.06
2I15	135	59% (80)	1.29	680	1.29	682.80
2HMZ	113	69% (79)	1.65	758	1.67	832.47
3IA3-D++	145	64% (93)	1.68	800	1.78	1012.46
2MHB	141	73% (104)	1.79	1120	1.78	1104.50
4MBN	153	80% (123)	1.93	1420	1.91	1346.46
2O9D	234	71% (167)	1.36	1290	1.36	1319.61
4E4V	485	63% (310)	1.48	2690	1.47	2599.31
2YNS	490	64% (314)	1.53	2759	1.55	2772.50
4BA3	496	64% (319)	1.55	2839	1.56	2845.84

Note: +3IA3 chain A, ++3IA3 chain D, and the rest of the above proteins are chain A if there are more than one chain.

The diffusion coefficient (k/D) is then plotted versus the number of helices (Figure 2) which then gave the best fit linear equation:

$$y = 74.076x + 356 \quad (R^2 = 0.9843) \tag{10}$$

where y is the diffusion coefficient (k/D) and x is the number of helices.

From Figure 2 and from the data in Table 1, proteins with about 65% alpha-helical segments fit closely with the plot of Eq. (10) for the diffusion coefficient of alpha-helical protein in aqueous solvents. The empirical formula,

$$k/D \approx y + (\%alpha - 65)y$$
$$= 74.076x + 356 + (\%alpha - 65)(74.076x + 356), \tag{11}$$

seems handy in predicting the diffusion coefficient. The simulated values and the predicted values for the diffusion coefficient k/D of proteins are given in Table 2.

5. Conclusion

In modeling α-helical proteins via the winding probability, Eq. (5), it was shown that an empirical formula Eq. (10) facilitates the determination of ν and k/D. Using

Eq. (5) and the simulation method, it was also shown that as the length of the biopolymer increases, the values of the diffusion coefficient D decreases which agrees with experimental data.

Acknowledgments

W. I. B. acknowledges support from the Department of Science and Technology-ASTHRDP.

References

1. H. P. Aringa, Analytical Modeling of Biopolymer Conformations: A White Noise Functional Approach, Ph.D. Dissertation, Mindanao State University-Iligan Institute of Technology (MSU-IIT, 2011).
2. H. P. Aringa, C. C. Bernido, M. V. Carpio-Bernido, and J. B. Bornales, Stochastic Modelling of Helical Biopolymers, *Int. J. Mod. Phys. Conf. Ser.* **17**, 73–76 (2012).
3. C. C. Bernido and M. V. Carpio-Bernido, White Noise Analysis: Some Applications in Complex Systems, Biophysics, and Quantum Mechanics, *Int. J. Mod. Phys. B* **26**, 1230014 (2012).
4. K. Dill, K. Ghosh and J. Schmit, Physical Limits of Cells and Proteomes, *Proc. Natl. Acad. Sci.* **44**, 108, (2011).
5. J. Wang and T. Hou, Application of Molecular Dynamics Simulations in Molecular Property Prediction II: Diffusion Coefficient. *J. Compu Chem.* **32**, 16 (2011).
6. S. F. Edwards, *Proc. Phys. Soc. London,* **91**, 513–519 (1967);
7. S. Prager and H. L. Frisch, *J. Chem. Phys.* **46**, 1475 (1967).
8. L. S. Schulman, *Techniques and Applications of Path Integration* (Wiley, New York, 1981).
9. M. G. Laidlaw and C. M. DeWitt, *Phys. Rev. D* **3**, 1375 (1971).
10. C. C. Bernido and M. V. Carpio-Bernido, *J. Math. Phys.* **43**, 1728–1736 (2002).
11. C. C. Bernido and A. Inomata, *J. Math. Phys.* **22**, 715 (1981).
12. I. S. Gradshteyn and I. M. Ryzhik, *Table of Integrals, Series, and Products,* 5th ed. (Academic Press, San Diego, 1994).
13. M. Abramowitz and I. A. Stegun, *Handbook of Mathematical Functions with Formulas, Graphs, and Mathematical Tables* (National Bureau of Standards, Washington D. C., 1972).
14. See, e.g. Table 2, S. Papadopoulos, K.D. Jurgens and G. Gros, Protein Diffusion in Living Skeletal Muscle Fibers: Dependence on Protein Size, Fiber Type, and Contraction, *Biophys. J.*, 79, 2084–2094 (2000).

7th Jagna International Workshop (2014)
International Journal of Modern Physics: Conference Series
Vol. 36 (2015) 1597001 (3 pages)
© World Scientific Publishing Company
DOI: 10.1142/S2010194515970010

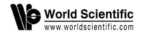

Subject Index

7th Jagna International Workshop (2014)
International Journal of Modern Physics: Conference Series
Vol. 36 (2015) 1599001 (1 page)
© World Scientific Publishing Company
DOI: 10.1142/S2010194515990013

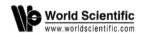

Author Index

A
Aringa, H. P., 1560018

B
Barredo, W. I., 1560018
Bernido, C. C., 1560006, 1560018
Bornales, J. B., 1560016, 1560017, 1560018

C
Carpio-Bernido, M. V., 1560006
Choo, K. Y., 1560008
Confesor, M. N. P., 1560009, 1560010

D
da Silva, J. L., 1560003

E
Eab, C. H., 1560001
Escobido, M.G. O., 1560012
Esguerra, J. P. H., 1560014, 1560015

G
Gemao, B. V., 1560017
Guang, H.G., 1560011

H
Hatano, N., 1560012

K
Khoon, L. K., 1560011

L
Lacubtan, R. J. L., 1560010
Legara, E. F., 1560011
Lim, S. C., 1560001

M
Metzler, R., 1560007
Monterola, C., 1560011
Muniandy, S. V., 1560008

N
Nayga, M. M., 1560015
Niere, H. M., 1560013

S
Sambo, J. P. B., 1560017
Shevchenko, G., 1560002, 1560004
Streit, L., 1560016
Suryawan, H. P., 1560005

T
Tare, J. D., 1560014

V
Viitasaari, L., 1560004